"ADHD challenges a child and also a family; *The Family ADHD Solution* balances an expert approach to the science of understanding, managing, and living with ADHD with practical, evidence-based, and sympathetic strategies for the whole family. Dr. Bertin will help parents and children cope, understand what is happening, and live and learn together from one day to the next."

—Perri Klass, MD, author of *Treatment Kind and Fair:*
Letters to a Young Doctor

"Mark Bertin has written an insightful guide to help families approach the challenges of attentional difficulties with a mindful approach. While 'attention deficit' refers to a complex set of dysfunctions in much more than the focus of attention, it fills families with a wide array of issues. To support the ever-stressful journey, the author takes the important but often forgotten stance that caregivers need their own deep understanding and self-care in order to function well and offer the optimal help to their children.... Research has suggested that learning to be mindfully aware can help reduce stress, focus the mind, keep emotions balanced, and even improve your immune function.... So why not take the small amount of time to read this wonderful book and prepare yourself and your family well for the challenges ahead?"

—Daniel J. Siegel, MD, author of *Mindsight*
and *Parenting from the Inside Out*

"An excellent guide for families with children with ADHD. Mark Bertin not only explains the science behind how ADHD affects the brain but also provides real tools and techniques for parents to both help their children succeed at home and academically, as well as restore balance to their lives."

—Edward Hallowell, MD, author of *Driven to Distraction*

"*The Family ADHD Solution* by Mark Bertin jumps to the top of my book list for families living with ADHD. It captures the science and the human story of ADHD with clarity and specifics—and offers the first real approach to parenting a child with ADHD that doesn't blame the child or the parent. This book fills a gaping hole in the ADHD parenting bookshelf."

—Candida Fink, MD, author of *The Ups and Downs of*
Raising a Bipolar Child

"I highly recommend this book. It's excellent, comprehensive coverage of practical information linked to scholarly research will help parents better understand and cope with the expectable challenges of parenting a youngster with ADHD."

—Norman Brier, professor of Pediatrics and Psychiatry and the Behavioral
Sciences, Albert Einstein College of Medicine

"With compassion and insight, in language that is easy to understand, Dr. Bertin has taken on the task of explaining ADHD to families struggling to make sense of this difficult topic.... A book that should be on the bookshelf of every parent and grandparent of a child with ADHD."

—Robert Marion, MD, director of the Children's Evaluation and
Rehabilitation Center at Albert Einstein College of Medicine
and author of *Genetic Rounds*

The Family ADHD Solution

A SCIENTIFIC APPROACH TO MAXIMIZING YOUR CHILD'S ATTENTION AND MINIMIZING PARENTAL STRESS

MARK BERTIN, MD

palgrave
macmillan

First published in 2011 by
PALGRAVE MACMILLAN®
in the United States—a division of St. Martin's Press LLC,
175 Fifth Avenue, New York, NY 10010.

Where this book is distributed in the UK, Europe and the rest of the world,
this is by Palgrave Macmillan, a division of Macmillan Publishers Limited,
registered in England, company number 785998, of Houndmills, Basingstoke,
Hampshire RG21 6XS.

Palgrave Macmillan is the global academic imprint of the above companies and
has companies and representatives throughout the world.

Palgrave® and Macmillan® are registered trademarks in the United States, the
United Kingdom, Europe and other countries.

ISBN: 978–0–230–10505–8

Library of Congress Cataloging-in-Publication Data

Bertin, Mark.
    The family ADHD solution : a scientific approach to maximizing your
child's attention and minimizing parental stress / Mark Bertin.
        p. cm.
    Includes bibliographical references and index.
    ISBN 978–0–230–10505–8
    1. Attention-deficit hyperactivity disorder—Popular works. I. Title.

RH506.H9B49 2011
618.92'8589—dc22   2010026236

A catalogue record of the book is available from the British Library.

Design by Newgen Imaging Systems (P) Ltd., Chennai, India.

First edition: February 2011

10 9 8 7 6 5 4 3 2 1

Printed in the United States of America.

For my wife Elizabeth, who was endlessly supportive and intricately involved throughout this project.
And in memory of my father.

Contents

Acknowledgments   ix

Introduction: A Thoughtful Approach to ADHD   1

Part I   ADHD: A Practical Guide

Chapter 1   ADHD, Parenting, and the Brain   9
Chapter 2   The Path to Diagnosis   21
Chapter 3   ADHD Beneath the Surface   39

Part II   Mindfulness in ADHD Care

Chapter 4   Attention Training and the Brain   51
Chapter 5   The Science of Mindfulness   71
Chapter 6   Taking Care of Yourself: Mindfulness in Action   87

Part III   Promoting Well-Being: Comprehensive Support for Families and Children

Chapter 7   Behavior: Avoiding the "No, David" Approach   125
Chapter 8   Education: Rallying the Team   157
Chapter 9   Medical Options for ADHD   177
Chapter 10 Supporting the Whole Family   201

Suggested Resources   207
Notes   209
Index   223

Acknowledgments

I am lucky to have many people to thank. Several people graciously read all or part of early versions of this book, including Natalie Baker, Cathleen Bell, Norman Brier, Candida Fink, Jill Green, Marion Katzive, Bob Marion, Jorge Pedraza, Amy Saltzman, and David Wortman. Your guidance and advice was immeasurably helpful. Also thanks to Joanna Faraday, Carol Mann, my editor Luba Ostashevsky, Debbie Mead, Elena Rover, Steve Salzinger, and Debbie Yost, for their generous assistance in getting me from an idea to a book. To my friend and colleague Dr. Lidia Zylowska for her insight, inspiration, and collaboration over the last several years regarding the science and application of mindfulness in ADHD care. Thanks to all my close friends and teachers who led me here, of whom there are, to my great fortune, too many to list. And for my family again, who sustained me through all the time and energy that writing and editing took, and my spectacularly caring and insightful parents (all three of them).

INTRODUCTION

A Thoughtful Approach to ADHD

Parents of children with attention deficit hyperactivity disorder (ADHD) often come into my office exhausted. They have been scrambling to figure out why their children keep getting into trouble at school—or, maybe instead, why their bright, well-behaved youngsters cannot keep their grades up. Managing their kids' behavior is frustrating enough, but then they start to hear from friends, family, or educators that ADHD is not real, or that blame should be placed on parents or simply on our busy world. They may have received a diagnosis followed by disjointed advice about what to do next. I see it over and over again—tired parents, strained family relationships and marriages, escalating academic difficulties, and families left adrift because the reality of ADHD has been made unnecessarily confusing.

When a parent feels like they're at the end of their rope, an ADHD diagnosis has the potential to give them hope that there is a definable, manageable problem at home. But then a grandmother or a teacher or a close friend steers them in a different direction. *Attention problems? No way, she's such a good kid, it cannot be ADHD. ADHD is not real; where was it when we were kids? He's lazy; you need to get him to try harder.* These are some of the common myths that lead parents astray.

I often see a spark of recognition in weary and worried parents when we discuss ADHD. Their body language changes while they visibly experience relief. "You mean ADHD *is* real?" they might ask. "This isn't anyone's fault? We can do something about it?" It's a liberating feeling that I witness day in and day out as we clear the air of

ADHD misinformation so we can begin to help their child—and their whole family.

During my first years of medical training, I felt off balance, not in control of my life, and overwhelmed by my experience, much like many parents I now see. Of course, every job has its stresses—especially parenting a child with ADHD—and we have all had similar experiences when something rattles us, or life gets too busy for a stretch, or something truly "bad" happens.

One day during my residency, I was handed a new mental tool to keep my head above water. During a lunch break, a senior pediatric physician led us residents through an exercise. We spent fifteen minutes or so counting and focusing on our breaths, all while not worrying about patient decisions, being on call, or life in general. The first step toward relief was that easy. I felt more relaxed, and though an hour later I was immersed in the pandemonium of the clinic, I had found a new path for myself.

Throughout the rest of my pediatric residency I practiced this simple technique whenever I could find a few moments in the call room between pages, or by pausing to settle myself before entering a patient's room. The more consistently I practiced, the better I got at maintaining my equilibrium and perspective in the midst of chaos. Problems arose, and residency was still challenging, but I found that I was more focused on patient care when at the hospital, and that I also unabashedly enjoyed my free time without half my mind wallowing in work stress. These tools I had been handed turned out to be common sense, easily accessible, and fairly straightforward. We can train ourselves to pay more attention to our actual experience and less to the random, anxiety-provoking clutter that constantly fills our minds, allowing us more consistent access to our own wisdom and clarity.

Coincidentally, at the same time that I discovered these skills, a huge shift happened in the field of neuroscience. Researchers found that even the adult brain is plastic—an old mind can learn new tricks, and when it does, the brain physically adapts and changes. Two of the most proven areas of study in this field are those of attention training and stress management, which, it turns out, go hand in hand. When we can focus our attention onto our real lives and away from scattered or ruminative thoughts, we feel better and we can more adroitly handle problems in daily life as they arise. One widely studied method of doing this is through a program called "mindfulness-based stress reduction." Mindfulness refers both to a broad concept—the ability to observe and live our experience without excessive criticism or judgment—and to the specific type of meditation I had been introduced to as a resident, one that begins simply by training attention.

I am educated in traditional Western medicine, a field based on evidenced-based practices. My fellowship in developmental behavioral pediatrics covered aspects of child development, general pediatrics, psychology, and other related fields, but not alternative medicine. So while I was interested in complementary practices, I hesitated to use them in patient care. For many years, I continued to practice mindfulness and discussed it with a few of my closest confidants, not ready to share with patients these thoughts and experiences.

Then I attended a research conference on neuroplasticity cosponsored by Johns Hopkins and Georgetown University. A collection of scientists spent several days outlining research regarding the adult brain's capacity to grow. They discussed the proven benefits of attention training, the science of mindfulness, and, of course, neuroplasticity (which I'll tell you more about in chapter four). One after another, researchers from academic meccas around the country eloquently spoke about this cutting-edge field.

All in a moment it became clear to me that these stress-management and attention-building techniques are no longer "alternative." They are grounded in research. Hundreds of studies suggest benefits far beyond lowering stress, as the techniques build an overall sense of well-being and support care for anxiety, depression, cancer, and numerous other conditions.

I come from a line of New Yorkers, street-smart, ardent, and sarcastic, without a lot of patience for anything that seems overly flaky or irrational. Razor sharp at seeing through flim-flam and detecting logical flaws, my family has always been blunt in pointing out their view of the truth. Mindfulness takes that goal to an entirely new level—helping you see through all the uncertainty and chaos until you can find the clearest view possible of reality, and then discover humor and joy in the midst of life's travails. If anything, I've connected with mindfulness *because* of my background.

Children with ADHD come in to see me with their families—their parents are confused, burned out, and living with moment-to-moment stress. They are at a loss: *How come he will not listen? We've read every book and worked with three therapists and his school still calls every day because he misbehaved on the play-ground.* Parents dance around each other, alluding to differences in their child-raising styles as a possible cause of trouble. They feel trapped, like there is no solution, as if their child's future is already determined.

For years mindfulness has helped me manage stress, stay in balance, objectively problem solve, and generally feel more at ease. And traditional science has confirmed the benefits. How could I not introduce mindfulness techniques into my medical practice? No one needs them more than a family dealing with the intricacies of ADHD. As I've now seen numerous times, integrating mindfulness into ADHD care allows family dynamics to shift, parents to smile again, and children to learn new ways of relating.

Mindfulness gives parents the strength and stability to take control of more traditional ADHD care, facilitating a broad approach that considers ADHD's effects on children and families. Mindfulness does more than help with relaxation, it hones people's ability to see the details of life more clearly and to respond more skillfully when challenged. When combined with evidence-based ADHD care, mindfulness allows families to take a huge leap forward toward a happy future. You'll learn all about both mindfulness and evidence-based ADHD care in *The Family ADHD Solution.*

I explain the basics of ADHD in part I—what it really is, what it is not, and how the biological aspects of ADHD affect day-to-day life. Hyperactivity, impulsivity, and poor focus are, to borrow a frequently used metaphor, the tip of the ADHD iceberg. The bulk of it, hiding below the surface, is the emotional, organizational, motivational, time management, learning, and overall self-regulation issues that are related to deficits in a skill group often labeled "executive function." Without this clear-sighted view of ADHD, decisions become muddled and unnecessarily complicated.

In part II, you'll learn how to train your attention, cultivate stability, and face challenges with strength and a perspective that encourages the development of new solutions to old problems. This mindfulness tool box directly builds the mental skills needed to move past entrenched habits and beliefs and teaches you how to address problems with flexibility. Finally, part III reviews comprehensive care and support for ADHD and is based on decades of research regarding parenting, and behavioral, educational, and medical care.

One answer alone rarely covers all the complex issues raised by ADHD, and in sharing *The Family ADHD Solution* I hope to illustrate all the various avenues that parents can follow. A clear understanding of ADHD coupled with improved stress management permits parents to make skilled choices tailored to their individual families. And with that perspective, I have found that both children and their parents thrive.

PART I

ADHD: A Practical Guide

CHAPTER 1

ADHD, Parenting, and the Brain

You're reading this book because you want something in your family's life to be different. Maybe you know your child has attention deficit hyperactivity disorder (ADHD), or you suspect it. Perhaps a parent, teacher, or close friend has drawn your attention to what they feel is a problem with your child's behavior. Or you believe your child is absolutely perfect as they are—but you would like them to be more at ease outside the family.

Maybe your child has been acting out. Or they are well behaved but struggling in school, and no one can explain exactly why. Even if you've received an ADHD diagnosis and some kind of plan, life may feel out of control. Perhaps you're wondering why, in spite of doing everything you can imagine, the same behavioral and academic problems persist. You've read every book and followed the advice of more people than you can remember, and still another call comes from the teacher: Your child is brilliant but never hands in their work. Your child pushed someone at recess again.

Maybe you're not overwhelmed and you have an easy relationship with your child, but you wish that life could be easier for them. You're sure they have the potential to succeed without so much effort or without so much support from you and their teachers. You're looking for a different perspective, and there's a nagging sense that life does not have to be so hard.

The Politics of ADHD

Attention deficit hyperactivity disorder, often called ADHD or ADD, is one of the most common behavioral conditions affecting children today—and one of the most polarizing. Parents of children who struggle in school and have behavior issues are swamped with information—and *mis*information—about ADHD. There is a deluge of unsubstantiated lore about the most effective ways to treat symptoms that often hint that parents or society are to blame. You may have been led to think that if only you could parent better, your child's ADHD symptoms would vanish. Poof. Just like that. But ADHD is a medical condition—would anyone expect asthma to disappear because of parenting changes?

ADHD care has devolved into factions. Some people, ranging from doctors to psychologists to news personalities and neighbors, believe ADHD is a myth, nothing more than a catch-all label for badly behaved children. Others suggest to parents—often aggressively—that medications are dangerous and they'll turn children into zombies. Parent groups and Internet sites swear that only their particular behavioral or alternative option will work safely—and suggest that other choices are useless.

And to complicate matters, what is ADHD anyway? Some people say it's real. Some people say it isn't. But as a developmental pediatrician specializing in children with behavioral disorders, I will tell you that ADHD is real—*very* real.

ADD, ADHD: WHAT'S THE DIFFERENCE?

ADD (attention deficit disorder) is an outdated term and is now included with ADHD, with the "H" standing for hyperactive. Don't let it rattle you if your anything-but-hyperactive child is diagnosed with ADHD. Medically, ADHD is actually subdivided into three subcategories based on different symptom patterns: ADHD-inattentive type, which describes what we once referred to as ADD; ADHD-hyperactive/impulsive type; and ADHD-combined type, a combination of the two. It can be a confusing concept—in essence we are saying some children have attention deficit hyperactivity disorder, but without the hyperactivity.

Decades of research have defined what ADHD is (a specific biological condition) and what it is not (a deficit of parenting or a figment of our collective imagination). Nevertheless, a morass of misinformation has muddled the perception of ADHD in the modern world.

Sensationalist authors make broad claims that a certain lifestyle intervention will "cure" ADHD, suggesting that our modern culture is perhaps the cause. Or that like fragile flowers, children with ADHD blossom only when raised "well"—whatever that means. Yet there are endless numbers of well-meaning, hard-working parents raising children who battle problems with focus, impulsivity, hyperactivity, and all the related disruptions ADHD triggers—and it has nothing to do with anything that happened or failed to happen at home. Because of these baseless societal claims, parents often end up blaming themselves: *If only I could come up with a new plan, or figure out how to motivate my child, ADHD would go away.* Through no fault of their own, parents often become blinded to the straightforward biological facts.

Stepping beyond the politics requires a return to the basics, with a clear vision of ADHD science. ADHD is a medical condition in which the part of the brain responsible for monitoring behavior and thoughts isn't working efficiently. ADHD is far more than a behavioral or academic problem; it has the potential to disrupt relationships, lower self-esteem, hinder social skills, and interfere with many other areas of life. Only through understanding the underlying biology of ADHD and its effects on brain development can you begin to make clear choices for your child.

ADHD by the Numbers

ADHD is not a product of our modern society; descriptions date back to the early 1900s. More recently, various studies in the United States show that around one in twenty children have ADHD, regardless of socioeconomic class or location.[1] Other studies show this average, to be slightly higher, rarely slightly lower, but, it is always close to this number.[2]

Wherever ADHD has been tracked—in Europe, South America, the United States, and most everywhere else—the incidence is near 5 percent.[3] How could an environmentally caused or culturally biased diagnosis have such a similar pattern, however and wherever children are raised? It is unlikely that a behavioral phenomenon could be so consistent.

Compared to the general population, when someone in the immediate family has ADHD, their parents and siblings have a three- or four-fold increased risk of the same. An identical twin lives with at least a fifty-fifty chance of ADHD when the other twin has it, and most studies suggest an even greater likelihood. This increased incidence persists even if they were not raised in the same household, revealing that the tendency is genetic. Non-identical twins have a one in three chance—again, even when raised separately.[4] Even the fact that boys are several times more likely to have ADHD than girls points us toward a genetic cause.[5]

Through tracking ADHD in families, scientists have begun to identify genetic markers for the condition. Genes have been found that increase the likelihood that someone will develop ADHD, and others may one day predict responses to different treatments. Just as some kids are born destined to be tall, or develop asthma or seasonal allergies, some children are born destined to have ADHD. Genetic evidence continues to mount; a 2010 study found a much higher risk of chromosomal variants in people with ADHD, compared to the general population.[6] However, as dozens of genes influence brain development, there is no genetic test to diagnose ADHD (and there probably never will be).

Biological factors affect the brain well before the potential impact of home life or culture. Premature birth, fetal exposure to alcohol, or lead toxicity in early childhood have been identified as ADHD risk factors and all make ADHD more probable. These external factors also interact with genetics, as studies suggest that exposure to certain toxins causes trouble only when a disposition towards developing ADHD already exists.

So in spite of all the media-hyped controversy, when correctly diagnosed ADHD is a medical disorder like any other.

Brain Basics

The frontal lobes of our brains are responsible for what we call executive function—the brain's ability to think, react, and modulate emotion. Executive function skills, which are reviewed further in chapter three, act like the brain's manager. Through pathways starting in the frontal lobes, the brain watches over behavior and emotions, monitoring, motivating, anticipating, and planning. The frontal lobes also regulate impulses and allow us to pause before acting. They determine how we organize our thoughts. They supervise how we think and act. They manage information, help us learn from mistakes, and influence dozens of related abilities.

In both children and adults with ADHD, the frontal lobes of the brain are smaller than in the general population. Research using mental imaging has also found decreased activity in these areas when people with ADHD perform certain mental tasks, while in the general population the frontal lobes leap into action in the same situation. When there is decreased activity in the frontal lobes, the effects on daily life can be profound.[7]

Doctors now say with confidence that these functional brain differences are the medical root of a behavioral condition and the cause ADHD. The differences do not stop with the frontal lobes, as they involve much more complex, detailed findings in various areas throughout the brain. While research is ongoing, these pathways likely include regions responsible for learning, emotional control, motor coordination, time management, and other mental abilities.[8] Keep in mind, these findings all represent trends—not every child with ADHD will have each of these problems, and they do not define any individual's long-term potential. (For simplicity's sake, I'll refer to overall brain findings as relating to the frontal lobes through the remainder of the book.)

As you can see, ADHD is far more than an attention deficit. ADHD is a disorder of self-regulation and a set of skills called "executive function." The stereotypical symptoms of ADHD—hyperactivity or distractibility, fidgeting or daydreaming—occur as a part of these broader issues. When these abilities lag, as happens in ADHD, children cannot effectively organize their thoughts or coordinate actions. The manager is asleep on the job, so to speak, and a child gets off task and becomes disorganized and inefficient.

A more descriptive name for ADHD might be "attention management, self-regulation, organization, and planning disorder." Challenges with self-monitoring, distractibility, irritability, and memory influence all aspects of life. Unchecked, ADHD affects brain development, how children learn and relate to others, and other far-reaching parts of their worlds, and it disrupts relationships with parents, social development, and schooling. ADHD symptoms cause intense suffering not only for children diagnosed with ADHD but for their parents and family as well. Everyone involved deserves equal support from the start.

Parenting Children with ADHD

I'm starting to get it. I got tired of all the energy I spent pushing them to do what I thought they should be doing. I was upset. I felt like I shouldn't have to make a behavioral plan. They should always behave like they know how to behave, like we teach them.

Now I'm starting to see, maybe they can't. It's their ADHD. They're not bad kids. They try, most of the time.

They aren't behaving like I want. For whatever reason, they aren't. Now when I go there in my head, I stop. What can I do that might help? How can I teach them something new? There are still behavioral issues—plenty of them—but the fighting stopped, and we're working on it together.

⚮

Almost certainly, we want more for our children than just the absence of ADHD symptoms. We want true well-being, whatever that means to each of us. Well-being can mean a stable, comfortable relationship with family and friends. It could be an internal state of confidence and self-esteem, or maybe an ability to face the ups and downs of life with equanimity and resolve.

Parenting a child with ADHD presents concrete challenges. Endless energy is poured into getting from breakfast to the bus, or from dinner to bedtime. Your children may misbehave with other children, fail to listen to adults, or struggle in school. You may need to supervise schoolwork excessively, or hover over every social interaction. Your family or friends may not understand what's going on, and you might begin to feel alienated socially.

You love your children without reservation and still, ADHD symptoms may push you to be more punitive or inconsistent in your discipline than you might otherwise choose. It may be hard to imagine easy times are even possible. At home you might feel like you are doing no more than putting out fires.

Parenting a child with ADHD challenges the hardiest parents, as the effort required to watch over a child's behavior exhausts. Trying to maintain consistent routines in the midst of the chaos is draining. Children with ADHD learn new behaviors slowly, leading many parents to assume traditional techniques are not effective, or to doubt their own ability to manage their children.

While most parents recognize the value of setting limits, or have read about it in parenting books, ADHD itself pushes them toward inconsistency, further amplifying the behavioral cycles. Parents may set limits when they feel strong enough but skip them when they are tired or out in public, where the stakes seem too high. And managing all of these ADHD-related issues over the years—it is no wonder that parents report feeling less in control of their lives than other families.

Yet the catalyst for change is parents, not their children with ADHD. Parents have the broader perspective, and when they regain control, their children benefit. Parents are at the center of most interventions, whether they are addressing their influence on behavior, collaborating with schools, or making treatment decisions. While, the bottom line is the long-term health of a child, intervention often hinges on adults.

Effective parenting of ADHD requires both patience and vigilance. To teach a child with ADHD skills and change behaviors, parents must maintain their resolve over far longer stretches of time than they would with other children. Under stress, or with the wrong information, decision making is difficult—but children flourish when their parents remain open-minded about expectations and discovering new solutions.

A Stacked Deck

I hate the word "focus." I really hate it. My dad is always yelling at me, "Focus, Larry! Focus!"

⚬∞⚬

Many of the symptoms of ADHD—such as acting without thinking, getting off task, or failing to sit still—can appear to be under a child's control, but are not. Kids with ADHD experience biological distractibility and have problems remembering responsibilities; they don't intentionally duck chores any more or less than anyone else. When caregivers mistake poor impulse control for deliberate "badness," children may become marginalized—on one occasion in my practice, a teacher even implied a preschool child might be "evil." Any advice that comes from the skewed perspective that a child with ADHD is bad or unmotivated is doomed to fail.

When writing off ADHD as "only" a personality trait instead of a biologically driven set of symptoms, children and parents end up being blamed for the problems. ADHD is no one's fault, but many people make this assumption when watching the erratic, impulsive behavior of a child with it. Parents feel judged, like they should be doing something different to control their child's actions. Yet while parenting will certainly influence how ADHD symptoms are expressed, it cannot overturn basic neurology.

Most often, children with ADHD try as hard as they can—even when their behavior appears intentionally difficult, poorly motivated, or maddeningly inconsistent. They could list all the rules in the book themselves, but do not have the skills to follow them. As Dr. Russell Barkley, one of the world's leading ADHD researchers, has said, "ADHD is not a disorder of knowing what to do but of doing what you know."[9]

ADHD is as frustrating for the children who have it as it is for adults trying to raise them. After they've acted out, children may calm down and realize, "I'm not supposed to yell." Or once it's pointed out they forgot their homework—again—they make up a story to cover up. They know exactly what they should have done and that they've let their parents down. And then they find themselves in trouble both for not doing their school work and for lying.

Most children with ADHD recognize their differences as they get older. They may notice that other children are not corrected in class as often by their teacher. Or that other siblings at home aren't in so much trouble. Or that their parents are frustrated with their behavior, day after day.

In a 2008 study, researchers analyzed college student interviews about growing up with ADHD. Participants recalled "a childhood and adolescence shaped by feelings of difference, isolation, and misunderstanding." They said that, as children, they felt frequent tension around household responsibilities, academics, and peers. They craved understanding. They wanted to discover a sense that the adults in their world recognized their challenges and the reality of ADHD and were reaching out to support them and intervene.[10]

Children with ADHD have their strengths and weaknesses like the rest of us, and ADHD does not define a person any more than any other medical condition or physical characteristic. Some people are skilled at paying attention, some at playing an instrument, and some are adept at physics. However, a fundamental difference from many medical disorders is that ADHD affects so many aspects of life, including traits and mental abilities often assumed to occur separately from their biological roots. Supporting a child with ADHD begins with recognizing this reality in their daily experience.

Quality ADHD treatment must address this truth, while never eliminating or altering a personality, or limiting someone's skills. Successful intervention allows a creative person to not only have a radical idea, but follow it through to completion. It allows an extroverted person to be social and entertaining but respect other people's boundaries, and maintain their own.

Treatment needs to protect children's strengths and at the same time target where kids could benefit from support. Children with ADHD have poorly functioning frontal lobes. They require care that builds from understanding what is willful versus what is a neurologically based lack of a particular skill. Well-being then grows from looking beyond the stereotypical list of symptoms and instead focusing on whole children, families, and communities.

The Myth of Perfect

I felt like a complete failure as a parent. I tried sticker charts and time outs and yelling and not yelling. And still Charlie wouldn't listen. I'd explain all the rules before going to the playground, and I'd turn around and he'd push someone again. It didn't make any sense. I was sure I was doing something completely wrong.

༄

There is no perfect step-by-step guide book on how to raise a child, so instead we're left on our own to sort through the conflicting advice we encounter in the world. When a child has ADHD, the stakes for parents are raised. Where one child might respond to a quick reprimand, a child with ADHD turns around and throws sand again and again. Bumps in the academic road persist and become mountains, exhausting in scale. Instead of a single bad grade or a passing fight with a friend, children with ADHD encounter chronic academic failure, or struggle to maintain friendships.

Unsurprisingly, parents of children with ADHD carry more anxiety and a higher risk of depression.[11] They report feeling burdened by the decisions they face around behavioral, educational, and medical decisions.[12] Their marriages are strained—couples affected by ADHD are more likely to end up divorced.[13]

Extended families and people in the community may often seem judgmental. They might assume a parent could control their child's behavior if only they tried harder, or made better choices. Stories on television or in magazines raise doubts that biologically driven behavioral problems like ADHD exist. The politics of child development breed uncertainty in parents, leaving them adrift and taxing their sense of control.

Dealing with ADHD, you may wonder why life has to be so complicated. It may be immensely frustrating to observe your child repeating his self-destructive behavior. You know, for sure, that if he could stop standing so close to his peers, or stop knocking over their toys, he would get along better. But the situation is equally frustrating for your child. It's not like he wandered up to the sand box thinking, "How can I alienate everyone, all at once?" However unskilled his approach may seem, he's trying to find peace of mind, just like you are.

◦∞◦

Reading this, you might think to yourself, "I've been doing it wrong." Or you might find yourself comparing all the advice that follows in this book to what you have done in the past. When you started your family, you may have had a picture of what everything would be like. You may have expected that your family members would act in a certain way, or that by working hard you and your kids would succeed all the time. Most of us recognize this inner voice that escalates our fear that we're not parenting "the right way."

There may be times in life when "perfect" makes sense. Driving somewhere, we want to take the right route, make the right turns, and get there. But despite our best intentions, we will, at some point, get absolutely and completely lost. How do we respond emotionally when we make a wrong turn? How can we separate our emotions from the fact that we messed up?

Most of life is not like driving, it's like baseball. The best hitters bat .300. Seven out of ten times they are out. They practice and refine, strive to improve—but never get much above .300. How long would a player last who eviscerated himself after each strikeout? Not someone who was angry for a moment, or miserable after striking out with the bases loaded, but who truly assaulted himself? How long would a player last who, overwhelmed, stopped practicing at all? Welcome to parenting— you can't expect to bat 1.000, and neither can your children. Perfection is not the goal.

Taking the First Step

A broad approach to ADHD starts with a proactive plan to address the most obvious ADHD symptoms, and then continues much further. It helps children build self-esteem and healthy relationships with parents and peers. It helps you manage your own stress because under stress, none of us acts at our best. It helps you examine your actions and cultivate skills that lead you and your children to be adaptable and resilient. You cannot erase your child's medical condition, but you can make astute choices about what to do next, for your child and for your family.

Building your own strength and resilience as a parent benefits your entire family. When you feel on more solid ground, problem solving becomes more flexible. Destructive habits can be broken, and new options become apparent. Your perspective, and your parenting skills, can fundamentally change. With an all-consuming problem like your child's ADHD, these life skills become even more important.

Over recent decades mainstream Western culture and health care have embraced the Eastern concept of "mindfulness" as a means of developing these abilities, separating it from spirituality or religion. Mindfulness is often described as living with full awareness of our moment-to-moment experience, without excessive judgment and bias. It comprises a skill set that helps us focus on life as it happens, instead of becoming lost in distracting fantasies of the future, rumination about the past, or emotional reactions that clutter our minds. Practicing mindfulness, we often discover a sense of inner strength and calm in the midst of storms that come and go in our lives.

We train ourselves to focus our attention where we want, away from mental distraction and onto the situation at hand. This skill can be developed through a type of meditation that is about little more than focused attention—our mind becomes lost in thought, and we bring it back. The art of mindfulness is noticing our mind wandering, and guiding it back to real life and to a sense of balance, without giving ourselves a hard time for having wandered off in the first place. We try our best, our thoughts drift off, and we think, *of course I got distracted, that happens,* and start over again, paying attention.

While our children come first in so many ways, it is important that we take care of ourselves as well. Our physical and mental health benefits them. When stressed, we easily fall into fixed, habitual ways of dealing with stress, limiting ourselves and how we interact with people around us, and perhaps not addressing problems as adeptly as we are capable. So in the face of all the challenges of parenting a child with ADHD, protecting whatever small nurturing moments you find for yourself helps your children.

The long-term goals never change—we all want our children to thrive and be independent and happy. In the short term, the most loving and supportive approach is to take an objective, clear-sighted look at a child's skills and challenges right now, in this moment. From that starting point, an entirely new way of living with ADHD may begin.

CHAPTER 2

The Path to Diagnosis

In spite of what we know about brain structure and chemistry in ADHD, you cannot take a picture of an individual brain, or measure brain activity, or use any particular computer test and say definitively that someone has ADHD. Diagnosis depends on clinical judgment—evaluators determine that a child's difficulties stem from an inherent biological trait. While we lack a specific test to confirm a diagnosis of ADHD, as long as a child receives a comprehensive evaluation, accurate diagnosis is possible. Thorough diagnosis also involves digging for related problems, such as learning disabilities, anxiety, and many other issues.

❧

The Illusion of Over-Diagnosis

People often ask: ADHD seems to be so common now, compared to when I was growing up. Has something really changed?

Researchers have evaluated large groups of children, looking for a consistent pattern of over-diagnosis—children who had been identified as having ADHD but who actually did not suffer from the disorder. When medicine lacks a definitive test, the possibility for misdiagnosis exists. Yet these studies instead show that when children receive detailed evaluations, over-diagnosis is uncommon. People may be quicker to wonder if a misbehaving boy has ADHD than years ago, but there is not a trend of mistaken diagnosis.[1]

Looking in detail at the rates of diagnosis in the United States, *missed* ADHD turns out to be more of a concern. Parents who have been mislead about what ADHD looks like, or who fear the diagnosis, may avoid seeking care. And both cultural beliefs and poor mental health coverage prevent children from receiving evaluations.

In addition, smart, well-behaved children with inattentive symptoms like internal struggles with distractibility, organization, or social problems, often fly under the radar. Quiet and well-behaved, they fade into the background. Through a misunderstanding of ADHD these children with inattentive-type symptoms may never get evaluated. They end up stranded and without support, at odds with parents and teachers who miss the biological reality of their struggles.

How ADHD Is Diagnosed

"My husband resisted everything from the start. He thought it was normal for a child to forget his homework, day after day. Even when I pointed out no one else in class did, he told me that's how he was as a child. We all knew Steve was smart—his IQ is far above anyone else in the family—and he kept getting Bs and Cs. And my husband thought Steve needed to find himself. Finally I said, of course he's exactly like you. You've done great. But why let him suffer? You barely got into college because you were struggling so much. You were always in trouble. Now you're happy—but why does Steve have to go through all that pain?"

○∞○

While not overtly life threatening like asthma or diabetes, ADHD is no less real. As with any medical condition it stems from a concrete biological problem, manifesting with emotional and behavioral, rather than physical, symptoms. Even though we know this about ADHD we do not yet have a definitive test for it. Instead, we're left with a clinical diagnosis—evaluators attempt to establish through observation and a proven set of criteria that ADHD symptoms are an intrinsic and impairing pattern of traits.

The first step as a parent, therefore, is to find an evaluator you trust. Some primary care pediatricians are comfortable diagnosing ADHD, coordinating their evaluations with schools or other professionals in the community. As our understanding of the complexity of ADHD diagnosis and treatment has grown, general pediatricians are increasingly referring to outside specialists such as developmental pediatricians, psychologists, psychiatrists, or neurologists.

Even though the diagnosis requires judgment and is subjective, the research-defined criteria serve as reliable guideposts. If multiple experts familiar with ADHD observe the same child, they generally come to the same conclusions. But as much as evaluators strive for objectivity, differences of opinion will always exist. There is no harm in seeking a second opinion when you feel unsure of an initial ADHD diagnosis.

Another important detail for parents is that school psychologists are usually *not permitted* to diagnose medical conditions such as ADHD, autism, or mental health disorders. School-based evaluations can only suggest a problem and pinpoint developmental delays and learning disabilities. School staff sometimes recommend outside evaluation, and at other times assume parents will find it on their own. But when a school psychologist completes testing and does not diagnosis ADHD, it does not eliminate the possibility that it exists.

Typical Development

"We wanted to let Dave be a boy. He was rambunctious and always active. He's our first child, and we didn't know boys could be any other way. He was a ball of energy, and so much fun, but by the end of the day I was exhausted. I had to watch him constantly or he would run away. It wasn't until I observed his classroom a couple of times that I realized he was the only one in his class who needed to be watched every moment of the day."

✎

Familiarity with typical child development is imperative when putting together an accurate clinical judgment. As one key piece of the puzzle, evaluators compare the symptoms of a child suspected of having ADHD with the behaviors expected for peers. Many preschoolers are very active and have a short attention span for play. Boys may generally play rougher than girls. Only when these behaviors become extreme and cause intense developmental, behavioral, or social struggles should there be a concern. To call a behavior consistent with ADHD, it must be outside age-related norms.

Most humans will follow similar developmental paths to adulthood: They babble and then speak a single word and then start stringing words together. Children learn to roll over and then crawl and then walk. Still, the milestones that guide physicians and parents are not rules; some kids skip crawling and still end up walking near one year of age. Not everyone follows every marker.

Attention and behavior progress through similar paths. The ability to focus grows through predictable stages, from a two year old able to engage in a single activity for five or ten minutes, to a high school student whose classes are forty-five minutes to an hour and require the ability to recognize daydreaming and return to the lecture quickly enough to follow along. Social play with peers starts near age two with mostly parallel play, and then more interactive play near three. By school age, verbally-driven, imaginative scenarios between children become commonplace.

These areas of development do not always unfold through linear stages, and progress may even seem to vary across environments. While completely unable to attend for a piano lesson, a child with severe attention problems may still sit and watch television, or become absorbed in toys or art projects. As we'll discuss later, shifting attention *away* when engaged can be as much of a challenge as a short attention span in ADHD. But for social, play, and academic skills to develop, some degree of focused attention is required apart from utter absorption in a favorite activity.

Individual traits and personalities are part of the spice of life. Behavioral milestones are by nature much looser than other areas of development (such as language or motor skills), but some children differ clearly from peers. I might encounter in my practice a preschooler who never stops moving long enough to maintain a social interaction; or a four year old who cannot sit long enough to read a book, to play with a friend, or maintain a healthy interaction with a parent; or a seven year old who is a constant danger to himself. When differences interfere with relationships, development, or learning, they may require focused intervention.

Who Has ADHD?

Parents often raise questions about the developmental differences between boys and girls. Some gender differences do exist in play styles and comportment, yet there is rarely a reason to write off problematic behavior because your child is a boy. Typically, boys are more active and aggressive in their play than girls, although not to the point of serious misbehavior.

Enjoying rough and tumble play is fine. But if your child consistently takes it too far, hitting or yelling at adults when corrected, it will eventually get in their own way. Other kids may begin to avoid playing together. Placing oneself in danger, overt aggression—none of these behaviors is acceptable because of gender.

Parents also become confused trying to sort out what is typical. The concerns raise a red flag—is my child different? You may not want to consider the possibility that your child is the one with a problem because you love them and want to protect them. It is also often quite hard to see your own child with complete objectivity. Yet seeking a diagnosis never changes anyone; it permits communication and allows targeted support to begin.

Part of the confusion may relate to your own experience as a youth. You may see yourself in your child. As mentioned, if your child has ADHD, the risk is roughly three times higher than the general population that you also have it, or had it. If so, it may appear "normal" to forget paperwork or always hand things in late, and to chronically lose track of time. Or to have a temper that sometimes alienates peers. Perhaps that's how things were for you. That was *your* life. But that doesn't mean it is necessary. You may be utterly happy and successful now, but why put your child through what you went through?

ADHD through the Years

In the past we believed that the brain stopped developing in early childhood, but we now know that this is not so. In a relatively new finding that surprised many scientists, research has proven that the brain continues to grow and change into adulthood. The natural development of the brain, and the frontal lobes specifically, continues into at least our twenties.[2]

As the brain grows, abilities regulated by the frontal lobes—such as self-monitoring, organization, and planning for the future—steadily mature. Young children, especially those with ADHD, have little capacity for future planning—that is, connecting the dots between actions now and consequences later. Most teens have only budding abilities to control their impulses, or to link present behavior to their lives in a few months or years. Even *without* ADHD, an expectation that teens will make healthy decisions while reflecting on long-term consequences ignores the basic wiring of their brains.

Kids' brains do not anticipate life in ten or twenty years. To an adolescent, a tattoo or a spin on the highway at a hundred miles an hour may seem like the best idea ever, right now. A teenager with untreated ADHD, therefore, is at even higher risk for common, risky adolescent behaviors because they have a delay in frontal lobe development.

The good news is that because the frontal lobe develops into adulthood, ADHD symptoms can improve. As the frontal lobes mature, many people with ADHD leave behind their hyperactivity and overtly impulsive actions. Others diagnosed with ADHD eventually lose the more common symptoms but persist with impairment primarily in executive function. Some people—perhaps a third group—outgrow ADHD entirely.

As I discuss further in chapter four, we now know that life experience continually remodels the brain. The brain's ability to evolve, called "neuroplasticity," has powerful implications for ADHD. It means that we may be able to encourage more optimal brain maturation if we can catch ADHD early. Several studies (which will be reviewed later, in chapters on treatment) have suggested that children who receive comprehensive interventions early have fewer difficulties later. Theoretically, early intervention may even increase the likelihood that ADHD one day will be outgrown.

ADHD Subtypes—What Are They, and Do They Matter?

Current diagnostic manuals divide ADHD into three subtypes, guided by two lists of possible symptoms. One list defines more external behaviors—being impulsive or hyperactive, playing too loudly, or fidgeting too much. The other group describes more internal behaviors—such as exhibiting inattention, poor organization, or carelessness, or having trouble keeping track of belongings or schoolwork. ADHD—inattentive type is diagnosed if a child displays six of nine internal symptoms in at least two settings (such as home, school, or work). ADHD—hyperactive/impulsive type is diagnosed if a child displays six of nine external behaviors (again, in multiple settings), and a diagnosis of ADHD—combined type refers to a child with six symptoms of both lists.

SYMPTOMS OF ADHD SUBTYPES

These are the behaviors evaluators look for when trying to determine a diagnosis of ADHD:

Symptoms of inattention

- fails to give close attention to details or makes careless mistakes in schoolwork, work, or other activities
- has difficulty sustaining attention in tasks or play activities
- does not seem to listen when spoken to directly
- does not follow through on instructions and fails to finish school work, chores, or duties in the workplace (not due to oppositional behavior or failure to understand instructions)
- has difficulty organizing tasks and activities
- avoids, dislikes, or is reluctant to engage in tasks that require sustained mental effort (such as schoolwork or homework)
- loses things necessary for tasks or activities (e.g., toys, assignments, pencils, books, or tools)
- is easily distracted
- is forgetful about daily activities

Symptoms of hyperactivity and impulsiveness

- fidgets with hands or feet or squirms in seat
- leaves seat in classroom or in other situations in which remaining seated is expected
- runs about or climbs excessively in situations in which it is inappropriate (or is excessively restless as an adolescent or adult)
- has difficulty playing quietly
- is often "on the go" or often acts as if "driven by a motor"
- talks excessively
- blurts out answers before questions have been completed
- has excessive difficulty awaiting turn
- interrupts or intrudes on others' conversations or play

The subtypes of ADHD are descriptive diagnoses designed to communicate where a child needs extra help, but in reality not everyone fits perfectly into one package or the other. We find that if children with hyperactivity have no signs of inattention when younger, they generally develop them later. And while many children with inattention lack any signs of hyperactivity, others fidget or act impulsively. Having more hyperactivity or more inattention flags particular areas of concern, but no one should be forced into a box. The label doesn't matter much as long as a child's needs are clearly portrayed.

We should never let the difficulties of ADHD define a child, so quality evaluation also includes a child's strengths. Regardless of subtype, for any individual a good evaluation defines and emphasizes areas in which a child thrives as well as those where more support is needed. While we focus on intervention and helping with ADHD symptoms, we encourage growth in areas that come easier for a child, for which they receive positive feedback.

⤜⧓⤏

Children with more intense behavioral issues often get diagnosed with ADHD—hyperactive/impulsive or combined type—when they are younger. Teachers raise concerns in kindergarten and sometimes even sooner. Symptoms of ADHD can be detected at preschool age, and parents often have a foreboding earlier.[3] Toddlers can show signs of excessive motor activity and fussiness, although diagnosis is rarely, if ever, considered before age three. Even at this age, impulsivity and short attention spans can be so extreme that they impair an ability to form relationships, or place kids in near-constant danger. One study showed that children who have had multiple emergency room visits for accidental injuries by age two are more likely to be diagnosed with ADHD later on in life.[4]

A preschooler who masters concrete skills like letters and numbers still may be falling behind socially, or having trouble developing self-esteem and confidence. For example, one study demonstrated that almost three quarters of the feedback preschoolers with ADHD receive from teachers is negative—not a healthy way to grow up.[5] Early identification allows for early treatment and helps prevent many of these concerns from developing at all.

Children with ADHD–inattentive type generally are diagnosed at a later age. Their symptoms are hidden, as these youth often get passing grades and behave well, but still do not reach anywhere near their potential. While they may excel academically, they require massive amounts of internal energy to overcome forgetfulness and an inability to manage their workload effectively. The biology of inattention may even be subtly distinct—for example, some studies suggest that different areas of the brain are affected than in hyperactive/impulsive or combined type.[6]

Inattentive children may sit quietly and behave appropriately, disappearing in the classroom. To overcome organizational struggles, parents may feel the need to micromanage homework, supervising each project step-by-step and making certain each paper is handed in on time. Kids can get anxious about keeping up, pouring effort into simply treading water.

While children with ADHD-inattentive type aren't as often labeled "bad," like their impulsive counterparts, there is a huge difference between thriving and getting by. They often suffer socially or battle low self-esteem. Distractibility and daydreaming scatter thoughts in conversation. They have trouble staying on topic or focusing on games. And since a diagnosis of inattention is often missed, children can stumble for years before receiving any assistance.[7]

Making the Diagnosis

While the biology of ADHD is well defined, there is no one examination or piece of information that identifies ADHD with total accuracy. In spite of what we know about how the brain grows and functions, the diagnosis remains subjective—an expert evaluation based on a set of criteria. Familiarizing yourself with the process can help you advocate for your child along the way.

There are four broad steps toward making an ADHD diagnosis. With them, evaluators strive to prove that whatever symptoms they find match the underlying biology of ADHD. They therefore check to see if the ADHD symptoms they've identified:

- occur in multiple settings,
- persist over time,

- are not being caused by some other medical or emotional challenge, and
- create significant impairment in the life of a child.

Signs of ADHD in Multiple Settings

A diagnosis of ADHD should typically follow when symptoms are obvious in different areas of life. For some children with ADHD, the demands of school exacerbate behaviors. For others, behavior is worse at home. One particularly hard or easy appointment with a clinician should not result in a diagnosis, and even a long visit may not reveal ADHD tendencies if it's in a quiet, one-on-one setting. Doctors or psychologists may observe problem behaviors in the office, but at other times they may reach a conclusion primarily based on outside information.

As direct observation in every setting is rarely possible, clinicians obtain details from teachers and therapists, taking patient histories, and using standardized ADHD rating scales. Commonly used checklists that you may encounter include the Vanderbilt, Conners, SNAP, or Brown ADHD scales, all of which attempt to quantify the occurrence of symptoms.

Rating scales help in diagnosis, but must be placed in context. Any particular teacher or parent or physician may unintentionally over or understate ADHD symptoms while filling out a form. As this fact cannot be entirely discounted, a clinician's judgment may trump any single behavioral screening test in reaching a diagnosis. Rating scales suggest someone does or does not have ADHD but will not confirm or deny anything all on their own.

Signs of ADHD that Persist

As a genetically programmed condition, signs of ADHD should be present over time. In theory, ADHD behaviors should have been observed to some degree through the years. Symptoms that crop up due to a crisis, a medical illness, a strained relationship with an individual teacher, or any other acute situation cannot be attributed to ADHD. At times, confirming symptoms across two different classrooms may be required to show that symptoms are persistent.

Even this seemingly straightforward, time-related point can be challenging. Our expectations change rapidly for young children. What may be considered appropriate for a two- or four-year-old child may no longer be appropriate for a five- or seven-year-old child. A child's fidgeting may have passed without comment at age four but might be a classroom problem at age nine.

As the level of independent work increases over the years in school, more and more children fall behind, clearly revealing their ADHD. In fifth grade students may be asked to write down all their assignments on their own, to decide what books to bring back and forth to school, and to hand in their work without prompting. Without extra adult help, the student with ADHD flounders—he is too distractible, disorganized, and forgetful to coordinate that complex sequence of events.

However, documenting early childhood signs of ADHD also is frequently difficult or impossible. Some parents may not remember early childhood well, and kids in foster care or adopted children may be without details of their early history. Adults may not want to, or be able to, track down this childhood information. Just because no one thought a child had ADHD when they were younger does not mean they don't have it at all.

Signs of ADHD Related to Other Medical Conditions

In pursuing a diagnosis, the evaluator also wants to make sure that nothing else is causing ADHD-like symptoms. Within medicine this concept is called *differential diagnosis:* What other conditions can mimic ADHD? Academic problems, certain medical and developmental conditions, and mental health or emotional concerns must be considered.

Instead of simply diagnosing every misbehaving child with ADHD, clinicians ponder an array of possibilities. For example, learning disabilities can make paying attention in class arduous, causing children to fall behind academically. If a child cannot focus on class material because of a reading disorder, that does not mean he has ADHD.

Several medical problems can cause ADHD symptoms, but there should be other physical signs or environmental risks when they do. Thyroid disease, for example, can induce restlessness and difficulty in paying attention—but not in an otherwise healthy child. Absence seizures (also called "staring spells") can mimic distractibility or daydreaming, but typically create their own distinct pattern throughout the day. Lead poisoning or chronic anemia may exacerbate difficulties with attention. And some studies suggest sleep apnea or chronic snoring creates ADHD symptoms, although more often they are a contributing factor, not a cause on their own.

Almost any mental health issue can cause attention problems. When overwhelmed and anxious, we have a hard time focusing. Obsessive thoughts (another aspect of anxiety) can distract children. Instead of listening to instruction they might be lining up pencils perfectly, or correcting work again and again. Children with anxiety disorders, therefore, may appear to have the inattentive type of ADHD—they may struggle with focus, miss parts of what the teacher is saying, and distractedly misplace their belongings.

To complicate matters, ADHD itself triggers anxiety. Living with the constant stress of forgetting what you're supposed to be doing, getting in trouble because of impulsiveness, or enduring the endless redirection of adults undoubtedly is anxiety provoking. And there are a large number of people with ADHD (estimates are as high as one in three) who have an anxiety disorder as well—the two are not mutually exclusive.

Many parents worry their child with ADHD could have bipolar disorder, particularly since there has been intense media coverage about mood disorders in children. The emotional fluctuations found in ADHD may seem like the random mood swings and extreme irritability that accompany mania or depression. Regardless of their cause, these intense behaviors can be indescribably frightening and upsetting. But mood disorders such as bipolar disease are far less common than ADHD, and careful evaluation finds that many children with these outbursts turn out to have ADHD.

A child may misbehave because of an upsetting or traumatic home environment or event. However, they may also have ADHD, as it can be a contributing factor to challenges at home, or in life. Many other situations exist that can mimic ADHD—too many to list here. While it is not your job to sort out all these details, you can make certain there has been a comprehensive diagnostic evaluation.

Defining Impairment: The Most Important Step

Impairment can be overt—failing in school, intense erratic behavior, or self-endangerment. It can be struggling with peers who, by the age of five, begin to have more protracted, imaginative play time together—which someone with ADHD may not be able to sustain. Impairment can be dealing with the layers of internal angst and anxiety it takes to manage to-do lists, to compensate for constant forgetting, and to cope with procrastination. Whatever the case may be, impairment means symptoms interfere with areas vital to the normal course of life.

Without impairment, ADHD symptoms can be considered more like character traits. It is, on some level, a matter of degree. Someone who is a little fidgety and active may be nothing more than a little fidgety and active. Someone who daydreams and is distractible is simply distractible if it is not causing difficulty.

Impairment also refers to various developmental delays. The frontal lobes, the part of the brain involved in ADHD, supervise the rest of the brain, and as we've discussed untreated ADHD disrupts areas of development including social skills, family relationships, and overall academic progress. The most important word here for a parent is *untreated*, meaning *without* intervention. None of this is meant to scare you—with intervention, families and children can thrive.

IMPAIRMENT: TOO SUBJECTIVE?

The concept of "impairment" is a point of controversy in the field, and in the future may no longer be a requirement for diagnosis. Symptoms of ADHD occur over a curve, from severe to mild to almost imperceptible.

Some researchers feel that ADHD can even exist, in its mildest form, without impairment. Others feel impairment is inherent to the condition. To many of us, the present definition which includes defining "impairment" works well—if there is no impairment, why start an intervention?

Gathering Information

Various medical and psychological tests can aid ADHD diagnosis. To date, none have proven accurate enough to provide a diagnosis on their own. Brain function is too variable; taking a picture of brain activity is under study, but not yet reliable.[8] Psychological testing may reveal attention or executive function deficits—or may not, even when someone has known ADHD.[9]

Computerized tests of attention can, at times, add helpful information. Yet the brain remains too much of a mystery to be defined so easily. People who do wonderfully on a computer test may struggle terribly in life with ADHD, and people who do poorly on the computer test may be thriving.[10]

While subjective, ADHD diagnosis is not arbitrary. The symptoms physicians and psychologists look for have been refined over almost one hundred years of observation and study. Concrete tests may seem more reassuring than expert judgment but to date remain less reliable than a well-trained clinician.

Seek a second opinion if you are not confident in the diagnosis—but when more than one evaluator agrees, or problems keep cropping up over time, pay attention. ADHD is not rare. And even if the behaviors you keep hearing about turn out not to be ADHD, reaching out for help is the first step toward resolution.

ADHD—or Something More?

Thorough evaluation accounts for the possibility of other issues that occur along with ADHD, usually referred to as *comorbid conditions*. Studies show that at least two-thirds of children and adults with ADHD have another related condition.[11] These range from such issues as learning disabilities to developmental delays to mental health concerns, and they often improve with treatment but can be missed if we do not seek them out. It is a complex situation to untangle at times, because many of the disorders that mimic ADHD are likely to occur side-by-side with it.[12]

The concept of "comorbidity" has redefined ADHD care, as we now know that treatment decisions rarely should focus on ADHD symptoms alone. Oppositional behavior is found in up to 40 percent of children diagnosed with ADHD, and a small percentage even develop actual conduct disorders, with behavior more intentionally destructive or malicious. Children with ADHD are more likely to have anxiety disorders, including obsessive-compulsive disorder, and several other psychiatric concerns. And studies show that up to half, and possibly more, have an additional learning disability.[13] Conditions including language delays, sleep problems, and tic disorders also occur at a higher rate than in the general population.

When reaching a diagnosis of ADHD, the assumption always must be that there is more going on for a child until proven otherwise. Comprehensive evaluation and treatment accounts for these potential pitfalls. And if you have concerns about your child that do not seem well-explained by ADHD alone, review these possibilities again with whomever is helping you coordinate care.

Stay on Target

Recently the diagnosis of ADHD and the discussion of related medical conditions has been complicated by the addition of two poorly defined terms: "sensory integration disorder" and "auditory processing disorder." From what we know to date, these diagnoses do not exist in isolation of other developmental disorders. Both sensory and auditory processing issues most often occur as part of conditions such as ADHD, anxiety, or, when paired with specific social delays, autistic spectrum disorders.

Sensory integration disorder sometimes describes children who fidget and like to move around a lot. Someone may tell a parent that a child "craves sensory input"—a complex-sounding idea that typically means a child cannot sit still. Other children may dislike certain clothing textures, or a particular consistency of food, or loud, crowded rooms.

Some children with ADHD, because of decreased frontal lobe activity, are physically active. As well, many children—especially those with an autistic spectrum disorder—may be overwhelmed by clothing textures, tags, noises, or many other physical sensations. Interventions that help children sit still or better tolerate various sensations are a great benefit, everyone would agree. But using the term "sensory disorder" may distract people from a larger diagnosis that requires broader care.

ADHD is also marked by difficultly handling information and managing attention—which sometimes gets described as an "auditory processing disorder." In a busy classroom, or in a situation where there are many auditory stimuli (like a party), people with ADHD battle to stay focused. Instead of hearing every word a teacher says, attention moves between random sounds and people's voices. Once distracted, people with ADHD find it hard to shift focus back onto the teacher.

Children with ADHD have real difficulty "processing information." When aspects of memory are disrupted by ADHD (more on this in chapter three), children and adults struggle to learn, or to organize their spoken and written thoughts.[14] They hear and forget things almost instantly, or they seem to learn but cannot retrieve facts from memory. Again, these "processing issues" exist, but not as a distinct condition.

When you speak with a teacher or therapist, don't feel overwhelmed by confusing terminology. Ask anyone using the terms "sensory integration" or "auditory processing" to be more specific. What behaviors are they observing? Is it trouble sitting still? Trouble paying attention in a noisy classroom? Aversions to particular textures or noises? By stepping away from diagnostic jargon, other answers may become apparent.

Not every child labeled with one of these disorders will have ADHD, autism, or something else, but persistent sensory or auditory issues are warning signs that a developmental condition may be present. Early intervention is critical. You do not want to focus care and resources on a small part of a larger concern, so if your child has been diagnosed with either sensory integration disorder or auditory processing disorder, discuss it with your pediatrician or another medical professional.

Getting Started

We all want the best for our children, but often have trouble seeing them with objectivity. We love them unreservedly, struggle with some behaviors, emphasize their successes...and may lose track of where they could use a little extra support. Or we circle the wagons and push back: It's not true. He's just a boy. He'll grow out of it.

For almost any behavioral or developmental concern, the earlier the intervention, the greater the potential for long-term success. Find an evaluator you trust and move forward from this solid starting point. You can begin with the school system if you like—when a parent requests it, schools are required to evaluate any child three and older. Or you can find a physician or a psychologist in the community to evaluate your child.

You make the largest difference for your family when you make clear proactive choices in seeking help. Whether your child is having difficulty with behavior, math, or tying her shoes, they'll benefit from targeted care, even if it turns out that they don't have ADHD or any other specific diagnosis. While no one wants to hear their child is struggling in any significant manner, objective decision making is the goal, and early intervention heads off difficulties before they escalate.

frontal lobe
of cerebral cortex

⤵ ⤴ executive
function

CHAPTER 3

ADHD Beneath the Surface

*P*roblems with focus, a high activity level, and impulsiveness do not adequately define ADHD. The name itself is too limiting—a short attention span or hyperactivity barely scratch the surface. Evidence indicates that
ADHD is caused by deficits in executive function, the brain's ability to monitor actions and thoughts. Executive function involves self-regulation skills
such as supervising behavior and speech, managing attention and sustaining
effort, organizing information as it comes into awareness and as we use it
in conversation or writing, and controlling and expressing emotion. As you
begin to understand executive function, you will have a much clearer understanding of your children's behavior and how best to help.

◈

Meet the Manager

While not always intuitive, behavior is controlled by the brain—neurological wiring determines much of how we think, feel, and act. The brain is
an organ whose role is to maintain "homeostasis"—in other words, to keep
our physical and emotional lives in balance. Our brain regulates everything
from levels of various chemicals in the body to states of mind, and brings us
back to baseline when our equilibrium wavers. Emotions and moods may
seem formless and ephemeral, but they have an underlying biology.

Within the brain, the frontal lobes act as the "brain manager." The
manager of a store coordinates the action of the employees and directs
purchases and deliveries. When the store manager drifts off task, the

store runs less efficiently. When the manager wakes up and gets on the job, everything runs more smoothly.

In a similar fashion, the frontal lobes supervise the brain, handling information as it goes in and out, coordinating actions, planning, and monitoring our actions. They monitor how we think, how we learn, and how we behave. They influence subtle concepts ranging from staying on task to learning from mistakes. Studies show that small or underactive frontal lobes lead to disorganization, poor impulse control, struggles with time management, poor memory, and emotional reactivity—all of which are symptoms of ADHD.

As we began to discuss in chapter one, executive function deficits are the fundamental issue behind ADHD—and the reason why ADHD affects far more than only school or work. Because their frontal lobes are underactive, people with ADHD become overwhelmed by tasks that seem mundane to others. Impaired executive function explains the related issues people with ADHD often experience, from emotional meltdowns to impulsive eating to motivational struggles.

ADHD is a neurological disorder that is not defined by a short attention span or impulsivity alone. Other issues are in play below the surface that affect the way a child with ADHD thinks, responds, and behaves. These issues aren't always obvious and can be hard to understand because they are controlled by what we can't see, rapidly shifting executive function tasks rooted in the frontal lobes. It is the rare person with ADHD who does not have a problem in some area of executive function.

Letting go of preconceptions of ADHD and instead seeing it as a disorder of executive function reframes a host of childhood struggles. The traits described in this chapter lay a foundation for an understanding of ADHD that will help you relate and respond more skillfully when you witness these behaviors. ADHD starts with the basic eighteen symptom checklist laid out in chapter two—but includes all the various issues that follow when executive function abilities fall behind.

The Not-So-Obvious ADHD Checklist

"Why should I have to use a reward system to get Mary to do her work, or to behave? She should do it because she wants to succeed. I've told her over and

over again, she should treat people like she wants to be treated. I can't use
reward systems forever."

⸘◈⸘

Executive function skills have been broken down in many ways by researchers. One grouping includes skills of attention management, task management, effort and motivation, emotional regulation, working memory, and self-monitoring.[1] Adapting this framework, let's explore how issues in these areas can affect the lives of families with ADHD, although no one child will experience everything described.

1. Attention Management

The "attention" difficulty associated with ADHD means more than having a short attention span. Shifting attention can be as challenging as sustaining attention. Moments of rapt, overfocused attention sometimes mislead parents or evaluators, even though they do not rule out the possibility of ADHD being present.

In fact, children with ADHD often have an almost excessive focus when completely engaged. They work for hours on an art project or sit immersed in television—and when it is time to end the task, a battle begins. You give them all the warnings you've read about: ten minutes until bedtime, five minutes, one minute...and then they resist and explode when the activity ends. Didn't they hear the gentle countdown?

Probably not.

On a biological level, someone with ADHD becomes so absorbed in a task that when someone else speaks, their attention doesn't budge. With normal attention management skills, attention switches momentarily over to the grown up: *Got it, I heard you, ten minutes*—but then it's back to their drawing. But with executive function problems, attention remains locked elsewhere—and a parent's requests don't register. A smooth flow of attention—I'm playing, now I'm listening to dad, now I'm playing again—is beyond the child's physical abilities for the moment.

For parents who don't yet understand what is going on in the brain, this seeming act of defiance and disrespect causes frustration to escalate. They often feel ignored, betrayed or angry. They may yell, or withdraw, or hand out a punishment. Or they may do nothing but simmer with irritation the rest of the night.

These reactions lead to a defensive, bewildered child who never noticed their name being called in the first place. They may soon realize they've done something wrong and become angry and defensive. Suddenly it's an even larger problem than it was.

The defining ADHD traits of distractibility, daydreaming, and poor focus also stem from troubles with attention management. Instead of being able to focus on an object of attention and stick with it, the child with ADHD flits about to anything engaging. Instead of noting digressions—whoops, off task again, back to class now—they remain lost in thought. Becoming distracted is easier for a child with ADHD than for most people, and returning from distractions is harder.

We all have our threshold for becoming distracted. For example, if you handed me a law book to read, I'd be struggling to stay focused on page one. In ADHD, this threshold for engaged attention is much higher than needed in life; it might take a riveting movie to grab a child's attention. Children often have an ability that falls at the extremes—either completely overfocused when stimulated, or unable to stay on task at all for less engaging activities.

2. Task Management: Starting, Planning, and Maintaining Activities

Task management refers to skills ranging from beginning an activity— stopping something fun to transition to homework—through organizing it and persisting to the end. Children with ADHD often battle over doing schoolwork. They don't know how to begin longer projects before their due date, failing to recognize how to break them into smaller parts. Their ability to manage and plan time itself is impaired. They cannot picture and lay out a project mentally, so everything gets left to the last minute.

Let's say an assignment due Friday is given to a seventh grader with ADHD. It takes a particular skill set to plan out the week: Monday I'll go to the library and start the reading. Tuesday I'll finish the reading.

Wednesday I'll outline and write a draft. Thursday I'll finish the essay. Instead, for a child with ADHD, everything gets left until Thursday after dinner. Procrastination is the rule for many with ADHD—not out of laziness, but because of yet another skill set that needs to be built.

Organization is a persistent, chronic challenge in ADHD. Some people naturally plan and prioritize; kids with ADHD do not. Book bags may look like trash bins filled with crumpled papers and crumbs of lunches past. Papers left at school need to be at home, and those at home need attention at school. When completed, homework disappears, never to be seen again—and certainly never to be handed in.

Lack of organization skills is a tough problem to outgrow. Even after the most intensive interventions (discussed in part 3), organization lags behind. Immensely frustrating for a parent, this is often equally overwhelming for a child. The paperwork or to-do list grows and grows, until the pile itself becomes the problem. *Keeping up* is nearly impossible—and without adequate executive function, a child cannot see the first step toward the larger job of *catching up*.

3. Effort and Motivation

Children with ADHD often appear poorly motivated, but what looks like inherently poor effort often develops from an inability to stay interested in a project and follow it through. A string of executive function skills is required for a child to persist in working on something from start to finish. Not knowing how to start or how to plan, how to deal with waning exertion or inefficient pacing, how to avoid distraction or stay on task, the child may lose momentum, and from an adult's perspective it all may appear like poor motivation.

Motivation in children stems from mastery and success, so eventually children with ADHD can develop true issues in this area. When children meet failure repeatedly, it is natural for them to reach a point where they give up trying—and for children, the task they are failing at may be something as fundamental as keeping a homework list. A cycle can begin where executive function problems undermine effort, which leads to lack of success, which leads to decreasing motivation, more failures, more motivational issues, continuing on and on. Building confidence in children with ADHD isn't easy. Kids will need external motivators, from parental approval to reward systems, to boost motivation until it blossoms on its own.

And while motivation may seem to be a result of our experiences and desires, research shows that a physical component is also involved. In one study, brain imaging found that the area of the brain responsible for sustained motivation may be underactive in people with ADHD— adding yet another layer to the problem.[2] A child may sit down with the intent to finish a report ahead of its due date for the first time ever, only to find themselves skateboarding again—and they have no more idea why than you do. Neurons in the brain responsible for maintaining motivation were not firing sufficiently for them to do what they wanted to do.

The ability to work efficiently—both quickly and accurately—is also an executive function task. Without it, a child who absolutely knows his math once again gets a C. He solves the most challenging problem but while rushing through makes a mistake with 6 + 3. Or he gets the work done, but it takes hours more than his classmates, or he skips over a section of the instructions and answers only part of the question.

Many executive function skills also overlap. For example, when a child doesn't have the ability to persevere, they become more easily distracted. And then, distractibility makes it challenging to maintain effort. In all likelihood, the actual neurological circuits involved intertwine. A broad perspective focused on the skills of a child is more important than teasing apart each individual thread of executive functioning.

4. Emotional Regulation

Little things that have the potential to annoy us happen all day long. We forget something at home we need, or the boss asks us to do something we do not want to take on. Hopefully, we have the capacity to pause and shrug most of it off. For larger issues, we can reflect for a moment and then choose a healthy response instead of stomping our feet. But with executive function problems—with decreased activity in the part of the brain responsible for filtering emotions—children react on a hair trigger.

ADHD may involve intense, moment-to-moment mood swings set off by frustrations and challenges. This biologically driven reactivity unsettles households, classrooms, and relationships. Each and every time something annoys or frustrates a child with ADHD, they lash out. One moment he is happy, the next he might explode in anger. Afterward, he calms down and moves on with life, perhaps no longer aware that he lost control. However, everyone around may remain quite rattled.

When someone is reactive because of decreased frontal lobe function, behavioral charts and external motivators alone will not solve the problem. Rewards help by increasing motivation and are useful, but they do not fix the underlying biochemistry. A successful reward system cultivates motivation while accurately gauging what a child is capable of.

Even though many of these behaviors are biologically driven, it does not mean you need to give up on behavioral systems. They may help with regulating extreme situations, such as setting clear limits about hitting. But as a basic point, emotional reactivity is more than knowing appropriate from "bad" behavior. Kids with ADHD may not have the capacity, yet, to filter their impulses.

5. Working Memory

Working memory refers to a broad group of abilities responsible for handling information. As you sit reading, or as a child listens in a classroom, the brain's ability to keep track of information before storing it requires working memory. We hold things in working memory first, deciding what is important, categorizing information as either necessary or disposable, and then storing it.

To later retrieve information from long-term storage, we again use working memory. In conversation, or writing an essay, we need coordinated access to what we know and then we need to mentally arrange it, paraphrase it, and get it out into the world. Working memory issues therefore affect day-to-day learning and productivity.

As discussed during the chapter on diagnosis, children with ADHD often can keep up academically until they reach late elementary or middle school, when work becomes more challenging, taxing working memory. Reading comprehension requires working memory. Details encountered from the beginning must be retained long enough to tie together the middle and end. Narrative writing requires retrieving information, creating a concept, getting it on paper, and then carrying it through linearly to its conclusion, all immensely challenging for many with ADHD.

Working memory deficits make mental to-do lists nearly impossible. You ask your child to run up to their room, put their homework in their backpack, brush their teeth, and hurry downstairs or they'll miss the bus. Half way up the stairs, your request is gone—they know they're supposed to do something but haven't any idea what. They may be acutely aware of the misstep. Inappropriate behaviors may follow as they lie or cover up with an excuse. Or they may feel awful, knowing you want them to do something. They want to succeed and to make you happy. They missed the chance, again.

6. Self-Monitoring

Monitoring of moment-to-moment behavior is another aspect of self-regulation affected by executive function, with deficits sometimes leading to fidgeting, high activity levels, or a tendency to get wound up and act overly "silly." Another related ADHD symptom, impulsivity, also manifests in many ways. There may be blatant acts such as hitting or running away from adults while out in public, grabbing toys without asking, blurting out answers, or even more subtle manifestations such as overeating. A want or urge arises for a child, and they do not yet have the capacity to pause and consider before acting.

The capacity to solve problems, another aspect of self-monitoring, also relies on executive function. To fix an issue, first you have to recognize that there is a problem—or which aspect of a situation needs addressing. Then you have to produce a coordinated, logical plan to address your concerns, and stick to it. Children with ADHD may fail to notice a problem exists, spend all their effort addressing a minor aspect of it, or, after trying something, overestimate the outcome's success.[3] They may develop a completely reasonable plan, and then find themselves unable to maintain it.

The frontal lobes also house part of our ability to learn from mistakes. Because of this, children with ADHD need more practice and repetition to learn than their peers. A child with ADHD may take several months to sort out what a child without ADHD can complete in weeks. This may frustrate everyone involved. It becomes difficult for parents to persist in maintaining a plan, and it is tough on children who want to please but are not able to carry out their good intentions.

The frontal lobes also supervise motor skills, so children with ADHD frequently have trouble with simple tasks, such as tying their

shoes and buttoning their coats. They may have trouble holding a pen-
cil, which puts them at risk for handwriting disorders. They may grow
up physically awkward or end up with a true coordination disorder—
which beyond having a direct effect on daily life may exacerbate self-
esteem and social issues.

The ability to monitor time often is distorted in ADHD. An adult
with ADHD might have a list of five things to do for the day, start with
cleaning their closet, and five hours later look up and realize, wow, it's
dinner time already. Or they may create a to-do list for an afternoon
that is impossibly ambitious, actually representing a full day's worth
of work. In the same way, children lose track, perhaps picturing being
ready by the time the bus arrives and then reacting with surprise and
anxiety when reminded they need to be out the door, right now.

Executive function also regulates social interactions. Children with
ADHD often talk loudly, interrupt others, or stand too close to people.
In conversation their thoughts may be disorganized, their answers distracted and off topic. Comments may seem inappropriate and impulsive. They may not formulate concise, easy-to-understand narratives or
explanations. All of which can cause social skill deficits both directly
and through lost social opportunities if other children pull away.

Reframing ADHD

For each area of executive functioning in your child, there is a reality:
Does my child have these executive function skills, or don't they? Be
curious, looking for patterns. As best you can, look objectively at your
child's abilities in comparison to their peers. Attributing ADHD traits
to willfulness or assuming they will simply be outgrown increases your
own stress, strains relationships, and may frustrate your child. It also
doesn't usefully address the underlying problem.

Children with ADHD are as bewildered as the adults in their lives
as to why things that are so easy for other kids come so hard to them.
Like everyone else in the world they would like to be happy, at ease, and
successful. They may begin to wonder, *what's wrong with me?*

They often need an intense short-term safety net, a realignment
of demands and commitments balanced with lots of structure to make
sure they learn and keep up at home and at school. And then they benefit from a coherent, long-term plan to develop their abilities and coping strategies.

Understanding a child with ADHD, and optimally supporting and helping her, means understanding how executive functions relate to ADHD. In order to offer compassionate support, build confidence, and create a plan for the future, the first step parents take is to sort out the reality of underlying issues present in ADHD, including all the varied implications of executive function. By holding onto these basic facts, you can appropriately challenge your children to grow while building for long-term success.

PART II

Mindfulness in ADHD Care

CHAPTER 4

Attention Training and the Brain

Much of what scientists thought about brain development in the past has been tossed out the window. They used to think that the brain stopped developing in early childhood; they now know that the brain is consistently rewired and reformed throughout life, including anytime people learn or practice a skill—a concept called "neuroplasticity." One of the best-studied areas of neuroplasticity is attention, which, as it turns out, is a trainable skill. Training attention helps ease stress and anxiety, because much of anxiety builds out of challenges with attention shifting—something scary grabs us and we struggle to focus away from the thought. Just like our brains can change, even our genetics are not fixed. Our bodies selectively express some genes based on our experiences. While we cannot change our fundamental biological programming—and we cannot cure ADHD with attention training—we can influence the paths our minds and bodies take.

❧

In a laboratory at the University of California, San Francisco, in 1993, two groups of monkeys were used to explore the brain's physical response to outside experience. While listening to varied tones, the monkeys' fingers were tapped by a machine. One group was trained to push a button when the tempo of the tones switched—thus, they focused on the sounds. The other was taught to push a button when the finger taps changed, so they concentrated on their fingers.

The actual physical experience—the sound and the finger tapping—for the monkeys was identical, but their brains were working differently. When the researchers examined their brains after the experiment, they made an incredible finding. The part of the brain that controls listening had grown in the monkeys who focused on sounds, while there was no change to that same area in the monkeys who paid attention to their fingers. Both groups heard and felt the same physical sensations at the same time, but focusing on sound caused the brain's auditory center to strengthen and grow. Where these monkeys chose to place their attention affected brain development.[1]

This experiment demonstrates what we now know to be true from a larger body of research: The brain is malleable and can change according to environmental influences. This finding has major implications because the same applies to people. Where we choose to focus our own attention affects our perceptions, our brain development, and our lives.

Training the Brain

Up until the last fifteen or twenty years, scientists believed the brain stopped growing and changing after early childhood. They also believed whatever genetic traits we inherited from our parents were our destiny. In reality, however, the brain adapts and creates new connections throughout life. We also know that just because we have a particular gene does not necessarily mean it will be expressed. That, too, can depend on outside influences.

The brain is made up of millions of nerve cells connected to each other by synapses, which are responsible for much of how the brain functions. A baby is born with tens of thousands more synapses than an adult. As we learn, we make new links between neurons and prune away unused connections. At age two, the density of connections is twice what it will be at sixteen. This pruning represents one aspect of plasticity, and is all part of growing up.

The brain is malleable or "plastic" in many ways. Anything we do repetitively eventually becomes hard wired. This is helpful for an activity like tying our shoes; we wouldn't want to think and plan where the laces overlap each and every time. But it also means that throughout our lives anything we encounter repetitively, including behaviors, reactions to challenges, and even thoughts can add and remove connections, physically altering the brain.

∽∞∾

Unfortunately, the discovery of neuroplasticity is being misused by people marketing 'educational' products, classes, and tools to parents. Parents shouldn't feel pressure to teach their children everything right away. Bombarding children with intense math or reading programs does not, in the end, advance their maturation or learning.

Development is sequential, and the foundations of early development are socialization, language acquisition, and emotional regulation. A steady progress of linguistic and cognitive abilities must be made before a child can learn to read and do arithmetic. Trying to jump the line—to teach academics too soon, for example—does not work. It also takes away from developmentally appropriate activities such as unadulterated free play.

Children require an environment that is stimulating, balanced by an emphasis on unplanned time with parents and other children to play and explore. Young children learn vital abilities—many related to executive function—from unstructured interactions with children and adults. Over-scheduling children distracts them from larger goals, such as social and emotional balance, that are greater predictors of academic and life success. It also can lead to excessive stress, which in itself inhibits learning.

Respecting neuroplasticity requires an even-handed approach, recognizing how much is too much, which skills to emphasize, and when. We guide our children by raising them in an enriched environment, giving them opportunities to independently explore, to succeed and to fail, setting consistent limits, and filtering the chaotic world around them. Our parenting influences brain development, but it is more like nudging a raft around boulders and through rapids on a fast-moving river than steering a motor boat on an open, placid lake.

How Neuroplasticity Works

The concept that neurons grow and develop new connections beyond childhood initially surprised many scientists. Yet we now know for certain that brains can adapt throughout a lifetime. For example, studies in dyslexia, first with children and then in adults, compared brain functioning before and after receiving instruction using an evidence-based multi-sensory reading curriculum. Researchers found that reading fluency increased as a result of the intervention; the subjects became faster and more accurate readers. A next logical question is: "What effect, if any, does that have on the brain?"

Part of the premise of this study is that people tend to use the front of the brain to attack novel problems. As activities become mastered, we delegate other areas to facilitate these rote actions. Much less effort is required, little conscious thought expended. For someone with dyslexia, each attempt to read is a new hurdle, so frontal areas remain active.

When these researchers used specialized magnetic resonance imaging (MRI) scans to look at brain function, they found the structured reading curriculum had changed the brain. Posterior parts used by fluent readers were now activated. These adults had trained their brains to use new paths.[2] A later study documented growth in related areas of the brain as a result of a similar intervention.[3]

Another small study involved playing the piano. Non-piano-playing adults were asked to practice a particular set of keyboard exercises for two hours a day. After a short time, brain scans showed an increased size in regions related to fine motor discrimination. Impressive enough, but in a follow up, another group was asked to *think about* piano playing exercises, and again, the same region of the brain grew larger.[4]

If thinking about piano playing can affect brain development, what is the effect of repeatedly thinking of something fearful? Or, alternatively, training the mind to focus *away from* fearful thoughts?

Changing Our Genes

Your basic genetic material is inherited from your parents at the time of conception. Within this information are about 25,000 genes, which contribute only about 2 or 3 percent of your total DNA. The rest is composed of what had been called "junk DNA," seemingly random sequences of bases not coding to build anything. Of course, 98 percent of the genome is not junk. It's actually more like an owner's manual for your body—the information that tells genes when and where to express themselves.

Your genes contain all the information that defines you—your eye color, hair color, height, and other physical traits. In addition, there are genes that predispose you to different conditions, such as hypertension, cancer, diabetes, and even ADHD. But your genes alone do not tell the entire story. Even if you have a gene putting you at risk for ADHD, you may or may not wind up with the condition. How and when genes express themselves make all the difference.[5]

Why does this thumbnail sketch of medical genetics matter? It turns out that our bodies sometimes can pick and choose the genes that come into play based on experience. The brain stops or starts certain biological tendencies, or one organ communicates with another, sending a genetic message: Danger ahead, time to focus on survival.

In certain situations, our experiences sway genetics in ways that affect a lifetime. Children raised under chronic stress—in extreme poverty or in neglectful homes, for example—"inherit" predictable changes regarding how they will physically respond to stress in the future, such as having over-reactive stress pathways in the brain.[6] As well, both maternal cigarette smoking and fetal alcohol exposure put children at risk for ADHD, especially if they are already genetically predisposed. So there may be children at risk for developmental or mental health issues, but whether or not they develop symptoms is predicated on what happens in their lives.

At the same time, no parent should ever be led to believe that ADHD is caused by how they are raising their children. Parental choices influence some, but far from all, genetic tendencies and aspects of brain development. While parenting styles affect symptoms, ADHD is a pre-programmed biological condition. As parents we can nudge our child's brain development, but beyond creating a healthy home environment and offering opportunities for growth and learning, much is beyond our control.

Training Attention and ADHD

One of the first questions about mindfulness and ADHD often raised by parent is: If we can train attention, can we cure my child's ADHD?

The answer is, almost certainly, no. The genetics of ADHD win. However, building attention is like building muscles. Increased strength and flexibility are possible. Numerous studies have shown distinct benefits of activities that enhance attention.

In 2009 Dr. Antoine Lutz at the University of Wisconsin published a study in which subjects completed a three-month meditation program. The style of meditation used was mindfulness meditation where, as mentioned earlier, one of the trained skills is focused attention.[7]

The measure used by Dr. Lutz was a test of auditory discrimination. In the midst of tones played through headphones, people were asked to track one in particular as it varied. Dr. Lutz found that people who completed the meditation training were better able to maintain attention to the sound. They also were quicker to notice when they became distracted and return their attention to their task.[8]

Another study explored the concept of attention shifting through a neurological finding called the "attentional blink." If we view a series of rapidly shown stimuli, at some point they pass our eyes so quickly we miss one. At a rate of one picture a second, we might notice picture A followed by B followed by C. At two pictures a second, we may still see all three. Much faster, we see only picture A, miss B, and then recognize picture C.

In another study, a group of adults was trained in meditation for three months. The group completing the meditation program improved the speed at which they shifted attention. In the midst of a series of letters, people who had trained their attention noted two more rapidly presented numbers, instead of seeing only one of them.[9]

While this study has not been repeated specifically for patients with ADHD, attention shifting is a fundamental difficulty in ADHD. These studies and others like them show affects of training on various cognitive skills related to this disorder. So can meditation be used directly to build skills in motivated people with attention problems?

In one pilot study, conducted in 2008 by Dr. Lidia Zylowska at UCLA, adolescents and adults with ADHD completed an eight-week mindfulness program. Dr. Zylowska tracked several measures. For starters, she wanted to document that people with ADHD could even complete a meditation-based program. Was it feasible? Could a bunch of people who struggle to pay attention to *anything* sit still and observe their breathing, or their bodies, or anything else for any amount of time? It turned out that most people enrolled in the study completed the program, including exercises assigned for completion at home.

Dr. Zylowska also examined several measures of attention. After an eight-week program people's ability to maintain and shift attention was enhanced and executive function improved. Numerous other studies since have shown benefits for attention and executive function skills both inside and outside the ADHD population.[10]

Mirrors of Behavior

The fact that children learn while watching adults is nothing new, but scientists recently discovered a neurological basis for this. We've always known that neurons fire in response to our own experience, but scientists now know that some neurons react when watching *someone else's* experience. When we drink water, these particular neurons fire; watching someone else drink water, they also fire. These neurons, appropriately, are called mirror neurons. Mirror neurons perhaps explain why sports fans experience such joy and heartbreak watching their favorite team, or why viewers get such excitement and agony out of reality television.

This hard-wired response system, reflecting what we observe around us, also has implications regarding parenting. Basic living habits form as children observe adults in their environment day to day. Kids are hard-wired to mirror experiences they see in their worlds; they are sponges that absorb the details of life around them.

We cannot escape the fact that our children learn life skills from us. Treat family friends and strangers with warmth, and your child is more likely to do the same. Children learn their own habits and go off in their own directions over time, but their foundations are built at home. And while we cannot model perfect behavior, we can do our best and then, when needed, model gracious handling of situations that haven't gone as smoothly as we'd hoped.

CHANGE STARTS HERE

Many intensive behavioral interventions in ADHD begin with a simple step. Parents are advised to spend scheduled time with their children every day during which their child leads the activity. Children need to depend on this consistent time with their parents. By using it as an introductory exercise in attention training and mindfulness, parents can enhance the experience for themselves and their children.

Choose one activity a day that you already do with your child. Find some play time or routine task, like walking to the bus or bedtime, and for those few minutes a day bring your full attention to the experience. Act however comes naturally for you, without striving for anything unusual; the goal is nothing more than to pay attention. Play catch, eat dinner, or read a book. That's all.

It's not so easy. Practicing this exercise requires breaking habits of living lost in your head, away from life. Note when you get distracted or off in thoughts like *this is fun,* or *I forgot to send that email,* or *I should plant more rose bushes*—and then let it go and come back to whatever you've chosen to do. If you find it helpful, perhaps focus your attention on details of the experience, the sounds or sensations or nothing more than the steps involved in the activity itself—throwing and catching a ball; serving food, eating, and conversing; turning pages and reading a book, or whatever else you have selected. Without tying yourself in knots, spend this time together.

Our lives are busy, and often we're mentally checked out while with our children, planning our next activity or wrestling with exhaustion. And yet so much of a child's behavior is driven by wanting adult attention and approval. For these few minutes a day, practice giving nothing else.

Teaching Children to Focus—and Beyond

Most experts accept that motivated adolescents and adults can train attention skills. The research has become hard to refute. Yet the concept of teaching young children often strikes a dissonant chord in our culture, and the overall question of how and when to start teaching children these skills remains open for debate. At the same time, the benefits of direct instruction are becoming clear in studies all the way down to preschool age.

Yet the broader concept of mindfulness has nothing to do with teaching meditation, yoga, or any other contemplative practice. Abilities like self-regulation, cognitive flexibility, and emotional resilience correlate with well-being and social and academic success. An initial question to address might not be "can we teach mindfulness to children" but "how do we best build the social and emotional skills that children need in life?"

So how do we best promote these skills in children? Certainly, studies with children have demonstrated benefits of direct instruction, using age-appropriate methods that teach self-regulation and focus.[11] However, mindfulness training does not displace the reality that cognitive flexibility and resilience, along with an increased likelihood of long-term well-being, all start at home.

Fundamentally, training children begins with practicing mindfulness as a parent. The foundation for teaching children attention and focus extends beyond any one parenting style or behavioral intervention. It begins with stable and supportive relationships with parents in a household that balances affection with consistent limit-setting and boundaries. Leading a lifestyle that models compassion, calm in the face of stress, comfort and familiarity with emotional experiences as they arise, and even-keeled conflict resolution influences children long before any direct training might begin. As well, emphasizing daily life experiences such as free play assists children in acquiring many basic cognitive skills.

It turns out that many traits that correlate with well-being over a lifetime, such as mental flexibility and resilience, can also be cultivated through mindfulness. Various programs that train these skills have been studied in kids. Researchers at UCLA have shown that preschool children are capable of following a mindfulness program in a group setting. According to reports from teachers and parents, children's ability to start focusing and to shift and monitor their attention improved, and they showed gains regarding aspects of executive function. They even found that children with executive function problems at the start—seemingly at risk for ADHD—experienced a greater increase in executive function skills than typically developing children. Other studies have shown benefits affecting behavior and social skills as well.[12]

Much of the art in these programs comes from translating the concepts of mindfulness and meditation so that they are both developmentally and culturally appropriate. Brief exercises of focused attention can be mixed with age-appropriate games. Yoga, which builds many mindfulness skills, is often integrated, allowing children a more physical approach to training.

Classroom interventions that promote skills such as an ability to delay gratification and flexible problem solving lead to a lower incidence of behavioral problems. Children who attend developmental preschools, which emphasize social emotional development and free play, may be more likely to succeed in school than those in settings emphasizing early academics. And strong executive function abilities are better predictors of academic success than early reading and math skills.[13]

Studies using various play-based activities show they are effective at building self-regulation, impulse control, and related abilities. Dr. Adele Diamond has been researching preschool programs that build executive function using a curriculum emphasizing fantasy play and other common childhood games. For her studies, she broke skills into three areas: inhibitory control (resisting temptations and impulses), working memory (holding onto and using information), and cognitive flexibility (adjusting to change). Her results showed improvements in all three areas. Based on these findings, Dr. Diamond is in the midst of research on whether this program may actually decrease the rate of ADHD diagnosis.[14]

A 2007 *New York Times* article quoted a child engaged in a classroom-based program who suggested that mindfulness is getting angry and "not hitting someone in the mouth."[15] Which sums up a basic life lesson—I'm angry, but I'm going to pause and choose an appropriate response. A vital skill for any child to have learned!

Stress Management 101

It was the first time I'd ever sat in meditation. It was really hard, but I kept listening and coming back to each direction—focus on the feelings in my knee, or my hand, or whatever else. I'd never realized before that I could put aside all those thoughts and worries I was having about what I need to do and what my kids are doing. I didn't have to pay attention to them right now. They kept coming back, and I kept moving them aside. And I felt more relaxed than I have in months.

༼ৡৢ༽

Whether you've been practicing mindfulness for forty years or have never heard the word before, stress will be part of your life. You will never reach a point where you'll do away with stress; everything in life changes and there will always be another surprise waiting around the corner. And there's no reason to eliminate your stress reaction anyway, because much of the time these impulses keep you from harm. A physical or emotional danger arises, and your body braces itself.

What we learn through mindfulness is to notice our stress cycles earlier and earlier. As we become familiar with our own tendencies, what situations create our stress, and how our body feels early in the stress cycle, we become more skilled at shutting the pattern down. We begin to recognize quicker what sets us off, allowing a chance to pause.

How you manage stress also affects your children. Stress is an interpersonal experience that affects you and everyone around you. Mirror neurons fire for something as simple as drinking water and as complex as yelling in anger. When you watch someone else get angry, stress hormones such as adrenaline and cortisol start to flow. You may not always manage stress the way you hope to, but the very fact that you are working on it will benefit your children.

Stare It in the Eyes

We spend a lot of time reflexively passing judgment on our experiences, adding mental layers to our already complex lives. This is great. This is lame. This is how it should be. We create emotionally laden stories judging everyone around us, from our spouses to the bus driver and especially our children. My child should be doing a better job. He should know better. He'll never learn to behave, he's just a C student, he's not motivated to learn.

And we judge ourselves. I'm doing a great job. Or, I blew it again. Or, I should know better. This running commentary isn't always helpful and can take over when we don't bother to pay attention to it.

Naturally, we tend to avoid things that disturb us. There are aspects of ourselves, our lives, and our families that we'd rather not deal with. They hurt. We don't want to go there. But when we see things as they are, instead of wrestling with a sense that something that already happened *shouldn't* have happened, we often find a chance to make assertive choices that promote change.

With that in mind, we can practice paying attention to what is difficult: My child is acting out. Every time I go to the playground they end up pushing someone. It's embarrassing. I'm afraid they're never going to have close friends. How come I can't get a handle on this? I'm pissed off and not thinking clearly anymore.

So you pause. You notice a complex and overwhelming wave break-ing over you. And then, you can start to practice letting go of judgment. The situation doesn't feel right, and no one says it should. But under-neath the acute emotional turmoil, what would be your most skillful response right now?

When you take a few breaths, you create some distance from chaotic thoughts and emotions. Bringing yourself back to your con-crete reality, rallying your inner resources, what makes sense right now? Is it time to leave? To enforce some discipline? To resolve that you will come up with a new long-term plan to teach them better self-control?

With attention fixed on a particular solution or a particular viewpoint, finding novel solutions becomes challenging. When you notice thoughts before reacting, you develop an increased ability to respond flexibly, to discover new options and perhaps to make more proactive choices. At times, below all the rumination and fantasy resides a simpler reality to address. If you try to stand up to an ocean wave, you'll probably get knocked down. If you know it is on its way, you might be able to jump over it, dive into it, or surf it.

Years ago, I woke one morning with a sharp knee pain that hurt whenever I took a step. I jog regularly, but couldn't recall an actual injury. An orthopedic surgeon was so certain that I had a meniscus tear that he scheduled surgery. To confirm, and to guide the surgery, he also scheduled an MRI.

For weeks, I limped everywhere. I protected my knee from the injury by hobbling downstairs, and I stopped exercising. I sat with my leg straight all day long. When I saw the surgeon again before surgery, I told him nothing much had changed.

But then the MRI came back normal and the surgery was called off. I had no meniscus tear. The doctor wasn't sure why I had the pain and prescribed a regiment of ibuprofen and physical therapy.

Realizing I had no tear in my knee, over the next few days I started playing around with it again. I began to see that, in fact, the original pain had changed. It wasn't exactly the same anymore. It was a little better. Over a week or two, stairs became manageable, and in a few months I started running again.

The mental state I'd created—I have a serious knee injury—had shut me down. I was unable to see an alternative. I was so busy protecting myself from pain, I hadn't tested the knee enough to notice the pain ebbing. A fortress of thoughts had boxed me into my belief.

Sometimes, out of fear, we duck our heads and miss the opportunity to notice a chance to head off a larger problem. Sometimes, without paying attention, we miss the chance to notice subtle improvements. There is nothing wrong with being annoyed or angered by something distasteful. But paying attention to our reaction allows us to break the cycle of stress and to remain open to the possibility of a different experience in the future.

Stress Creates Stress

Stress causes a concrete physical cascade of reactions throughout the body. It is our basic fight-or-flight response, our body kicking off a chain of self-protective events. From an evolutionary standpoint, it is a survival skill: *"I'm about to get crushed by a wooly mammoth. Run."*

A part of the brain called the amygdala fires. It yells and screams. It causes a burst of adrenaline and a shutdown of less essential activities, like digestion. But the amygdala has no intelligence. One scary thought—I'm going to be crushed by a mammoth—is the same as any other—I have a big math test tomorrow. Anything we perceive as frightening causes the identical chain of events to happen, and both situations kick off similar physical reactions.

Once started, stress perpetuates itself. Hormones excite the body, prepare it for action. The body reacts. So many of the ways you experience stress, from upset stomach to tightness in the chest to sweaty palms to headaches, trace back to the physical cascade triggered by the amygdala.

And then these concrete physical experiences lead to actions that cause more excitement and more agitation. And thoughts and emotions arise based on how your body feels. When your body is tense, your mind starts to wonder why. My shoulders are hunched, my heart is racing. I must be in danger. This then triggers more thoughts and emotions. And on and on.

What sets off the cycle? Once in a while, it's an actual physical danger. But more often than not, stress is triggered by a perception, an unconscious sensation that some experience is more than you can handle right now.

DEFUSING STRESS BEGINS HERE

Spend some time for a week or two watching how you react under stress, in the face of challenging moments. For the purpose of this exercise, observe yourself when stressed, without trying to do anything different or new, from how you feel physically and emotionally, to what you think, to what you say. You might reflect on what, if anything, you were particularly aware of while the moment was happening. As a start, notice any thoughts judging yourself, your kids, or anyone else involved. *I shouldn't act this way, he shouldn't misbehave.*

Either while you are still dealing with the situation or shortly afterward, write down for yourself what you were feeling in your body. Did you feel muscle tension, a dry mouth, tightness in your jaw, or nothing physical at all? What feelings, moods, or emotions arose? Did you feel furious, sad, fearful, or some combination? Where did your thoughts go? Were you at all tying the event into the past, or leaping into guesses about the future? What habitual patterns did you observe in your reaction, and in what you said or did next?

Attention and Anxiety

Anxiety is not always an overreaction to something worrisome. Anxiety instead can grow from the struggle to let go of a scary thought. Overreaction is not the problem; *persisting* with the disturbing thought is.

If two people are exposed to the same frightening experience, both feel scared: "Is that an angry pit bull running toward me?" A person without a fear of dogs may recover quickly—"It's okay, the owner has it on a leash. Not to worry." A person scared of dogs may be equally frightened at first and then ruminate about the experience, feeling the fear and related stress much longer.

Anxiety causes a circuit in the brain to fire, and this circuit is like a rut in the road. As you try to redirect the wagon of your thoughts, the wheels skip right back into the path they've ridden hundreds of time before. "I wonder if that dog is still following us. It's going to chase me down." Long after the event has passed, the thoughts and emotions linger.

A 2008 study showed this relationship between anxiety and attention. Young adults were given an increasingly challenging task in which they were asked to identify parts of a briefly shown string of letters. Researchers, using a brain scan, found that people with the highest levels of anxiety struggled to focus attention on the task at hand, instead of on anxious thoughts, especially during easy tasks. As the problems became more difficult, people became more engaged in the work and the anxiety center of the brain shut off. For less engaging tasks, anxiety persisted and interfered with performance; once attention was fully grabbed by the task, anxiety dropped.[16]

The authors concluded that these findings may clarify one benefit of mindfulness meditation. An ability to focus attention away from anxiety-provoking thoughts helps explain the increased well-being and lower stress experienced by people who practice mindfulness. Imagine the opportunity when we begin to separate our instant reactions from the feelings and thoughts triggering stress, or when, through an increased awareness of our inner states, we manage to reverse the cycle faster when it starts.

∾

Of course, it's impossible to never feel anxious or unhappy. We cannot find a perfect moment of bliss and then wrestle life to a standstill. Some amount of uncertainty and pain is inevitable in life. When we start expecting anything different, we set ourselves up for disappointment.

You're doing nothing wrong when you feel tired, unhappy, overwhelmed, or anything else. Whatever you feel is your experience. Each of us is doing the best we can all the time to handle our lives. Why would we do otherwise?

Breaking the Cycle

I had no idea what to expect. I'd never tried meditating. I thought it was probably pretty flakey. But it's not at all—it's logical. At some point you need to stop and pay attention and think about what's going on in your life. It's like when I was in my twenties and miserable in a good job and then one day I finally stopped myself. I was so unhappy. I was scared to death, but I switched careers. I could have kept doing it for years and years, forever. And it turns out that's all meditation is, stopping and looking at what you are doing and what's going on in your life. It makes sense.

⌐∞⌐

We spend much of our time in life lost in thought. At breakfast with our children we have a distracted conversation while hustling to get out the door. We're pouring cereal and cracking a joke and also planning what to buy for dinner or ruminating over a challenging meeting scheduled at work. Something rattles us in a conversation, and we spin off into anxiety or anger, and miss the details of what is said for the next half hour.

We drive while thinking about our job, making calls, listening to music, and not paying all that much attention to the act of driving. Or to the scenery outside the window. Or that we needed to get off at exit ten today instead of exit fifteen. So, we notice the exit only as we zip past.

There isn't much we can ever do, or should ever try to do, to stop ourselves from thinking. That's what minds do. But we never have to take our random thoughts at face value. While our beliefs and mental experience often feel etched in stone, thinking or imagining something doesn't make it valid or real.

Some thoughts are worth acting on: I need to find a gas station or I'll run out of gas. Some are not: If I run out of gas right now, I'll be late for my job interview, and they'll never hire me, I'm such an idiot, I should have filled up last night, my wife drove the car yesterday, this is her fault, where's the cell phone I'm going to call her right now...all these thoughts and reactions escalate an already stressful situation to new levels.

⌐∞⌐

In order to be aware of all the physical, emotional, and behavioral habits we have, we must bother to look, to pay attention. In order to break habits that make us feel stressed or overwhelmed, we need to be aware of them in the first place. So we need to sharpen our ability to plainly see what's going on in our lives.

We aim to break stress cycles earlier and earlier, to step away from all the habits we perpetuate when not consciously thinking or reflecting on our actions. The goal is practical, but hard to maintain—to pay full attention to our lives as they happen, without skewed judgments, and without getting lost in mental distraction. Pleasant, exciting things happen, and we appreciate them without expecting them to last forever. Unpleasant things enter our lives—and we strive to change them when that's a viable option, and to wrestle with them less when it is not.

Mindfulness meditation is one common way of training this type of focused attention. As we've seen, the ability to manage attention by steering our thoughts away from distractions reduces stress and anxiety. We train our attention to be where we want it, moving away from random mental add-ons. We build an ability to notice distractions as distractions, and return our attention to our present experience after each one.

Meditation also builds particular skills and attitudes such as stepping away from reactivity and giving ourselves a break when self-judgment arises. We cultivate an ability to be more present in our lives as they happen, instead of always 'doing' something, always on the go and never still or at peace. And in honing our ability to focus away from any habitual rumination over fears, thoughts, or emotions, back to the present, we offer ourselves an opportunity to live our lives more fully.

BASIC MINDFULNESS—FOCUSING ON THE BREATH

Here are basic instructions to begin practicing mindfulness meditation on your own. As you cannot read from a book and meditate at the same time, you can instead read the directions and follow them on your own later. Choose for yourself how long to practice, maybe between ten and thirty minutes, whatever feels most appropriate for you.

Sit in an alert and balanced posture where you're less likely to fall asleep or fidget. If sitting is challenging, you can lie down or stand. Trust yourself, and make whatever adjustments your body needs. Find a way to position yourself that feels awake, dignified, and comfortable. Let your eyes close, or gently focus your vision several feet in front of you on the floor.

When you are ready, put aside the book and bring your attention to your breath, wherever the sensation of breathing feels most obvious to you. You might recognize a feeling of air moving out of your nostrils or your mouth. You might instead notice the rising and falling of your belly, or subtle movements almost anywhere else in the body. Without changing how you breathe, without exerting any effort trying to feel relaxed or to control your thoughts, notice the physical sensations as your breath comes and goes.

Meditation often starts by focusing on the breath because, for most of people, it is a "neutral" experience, without a lot of emotional baggage. You are always breathing and wherever you are, you can use it as way to bring your attention back from wherever it has gone. The practice of mindfulness meditation at times can be little more than noticing when your attention has wandered from your breath, and bringing it back.

In practicing meditation there will always be distractions that grab your attention, anything from noises in the room to random mental images and deliberations. Instead of being swept into a stream of thought, pause when you become aware you've gone elsewhere and return to your breath. Let go of any sense of exertion, or of trying to "do" something. Each time you return to the sensation of breathing you allow yourself a moment without striving, without trying to get somewhere. You can, for a few brief seconds, be still.

When your attention wanders off—as it certainly will—practice lightly returning yourself to the present, letting go of frustration as much as possible. Expect distracting thoughts, feelings and sensations to arise over and over again. Whenever your mind has gone off somewhere else, come back to your breathing without chiding yourself for having "failed" in any way. Through the hundreds and thousands of distractions, release them and come back to your next breath.

Lots of judgment crops up when people start meditating, often about the practice itself: *I must look silly. No way, I'll never be able to meditate.* Or even, *this is great, I feel so peaceful, I'm sure it will change my entire life.* You may notice your mind going off your breath and think *I'm terrible at this*...but in fact you cannot meditate well or meditate poorly.

None of these thoughts or experiences are better or worse than any other. You may feel calm, you may feel bored or fidgety, and you may feel anything in between. You cannot in any way force yourself to be at ease or free of stress. Instead, you can balance the practice of noticing distractions with a letting go of expectations, sitting for a few moments and observing your moment-to-moment experience. Meditation, like life, is sometimes relaxing—and sometimes challenging.

Notice each mental or physical experience you have during meditation, and the related urge to act on it. *I've got to move, I can't stop thinking, I have got to write that idea down this moment.* While you are sitting, let the thoughts be. Some other time you may choose to plan, or discover something to fix that requires immediate action. Right now, give yourself permission to slow down.

As much as possible let sounds, physical sensations, perceptions, emotions or whatever else you encounter come and go without becoming entangled. You will never still your mind completely, or through willpower induce a particular state of mind. But by changing how you relate to your experience in these ways, you may discover a sense of stillness and stability more often available in your daily life.

Find a few minutes a day to sit quietly. Choose an amount of time that works for you, and then commit to it—thirty minutes, perhaps. Or ten. Or forty. You need nothing special to get started, but a timer may help at the beginning. Finding a quiet place away from distractions may be useful, but you can sit even in the midst of noise and chaos. You might not notice much of a change at the start, or you might continue to find sitting still difficult. However it feels on any given day, you are still practicing.

Like marathon training, there is no distinct start or end point with mindfulness meditation. As a runner, you forever refine your abilities and perhaps carve a few seconds off your time. You finish one run, go back to the rest of life, and do it again the next day. At the start, or on any particularly challenging day, jogging around the block or to the mailbox may be enough. Likewise in training attention and practicing meditation, focusing for even a handful of moments while sitting is perfect.

In the end, the point of meditation is not how you feel during your time sitting. While it helps to quiet the mind for these few minutes every day, meditation develops traits that maintain a settled mind and allow you to see situations more clearly throughout your life. As we'll review next, studies show that mindfulness leads to an increased likelihood of everything from an enhanced sense of well-being to improvement in certain medical and mental health conditions.

CHAPTER 5

The Science of Mindfulness

Mindfulness encompasses an evidence-based group of skills and traits that can be cultivated, with direct, proven psychological and physical benefits. Decades of research have demonstrated an increased sense of well-being, a lessening of anxiety, and a lowering of stress in people who practice mindfulness. It helps with specific psychological conditions ranging from depression to borderline personality disorder. Medical benefits have been shown regarding pain management and immune function, and for chronic conditions including arthritis, psoriasis, and diabetes. And concrete changes have been shown in the brain when people meditate regularly—increased firing in centers related to happiness and compassion, as well as beneficial growth in specific areas of the brain.

◦∞◦

For many centuries, the great thinkers of Western society have focused on conquering the world around us through science and technology. By contrast, many great thinkers in Eastern society have spent centuries refining tools that quiet the mind. Cultivating equanimity and wisdom through observing the reality of day-to-day life, without snap judgments and bias, is an end in itself. These methods, developed over centuries, are accessible to anyone. They are meant for use in daily life, regardless of any individual's belief about spirituality or religion.[1]

A New Perspective

Over thirty years ago, Dr. Jon Kabat Zinn developed a Western adaptation of certain Eastern practices. He called it "mindfulness-based stress reduction" (MBSR). This eight-week program separates Buddhist practices of meditation from their religious context. Since its humble beginning in University of Massachusetts medical center basements, MBSR has been shown to be beneficial for overall well-being and when integrated into the care of numerous psychological and physical conditions.

Dr. Kabat Zinn began his program at the University of Massachusetts in the 1970s. He asked doctors to refer patients whose bodies failed to respond fully to Western medicine. First referred were those with hard-to-treat conditions such as chronic pain or heart disease. Dr. Kabat Zinn recognized the medical world might be skeptical, and encouraged structured research right away.

From the outset, the results were clear. MBSR is now used at hundreds of academic medical centers and all around the world. Mindfulness-based interventions have crossed over into traditional, Western-based medical and psychological care. Even while researchers continue to examine the details, the perception of mindfulness meditation as alternative medicine is outdated. The overwhelming consensus of all the various studies is difficult to refute—mindfulness-based interventions have proven to be effective.

UNIQUE AND STUDIED

Mindfulness-based stress reduction (MBSR) is not the only approach available for building mindfulness, but it is one of the best studied. Other related practices, including traditional yoga, tai chi, and various other types of meditation have similar benefits. Mindfulness also has been integrated into forms of psychotherapy and cognitive behavioral therapy. Similar content can be found in many settings, but MBSR and its adaptations may be unique because of their accessibility.

There are hundreds of successful studies on this topic. The evidence points in the same direction across publications: Mindfulness meditation increases well-being, decreases stress, and helps with a long list of physical and psychological issues. In many ways the field of mindfulness has transitioned from asking *if* it works to an examination of *how*.

We still don't know for certain which traits of mindfulness are most important for individuals, or what aspects of the classes. Do people need to meditate fifteen minutes a day, or forty-five? Should classes be six or eight weeks? Can mindfulness be taught without meditation?

Research is ongoing to further refine teaching methods, and to offer people more sophisticated classes and advice. The process of adapting the program culturally and to different age groups also continues every day. But as a bottom line, mindfulness training does *something* that helps people live their lives differently. And for parents of children with ADHD, it addresses a body of skills parents need to take control of their lives, find objectivity and clarity in the midst of confusion, cultivate their own inner strength and resilience, and rediscover warmth and compassion in strained family relationships.

An Evidence-Based Approach to Health and Well-Being

The *Journal of the American Medical Association (JAMA)* is one of the more established medical journals. Its standards are high. In 2009 *JAMA* published a study showing that mindfulness relieves burnout and increases empathy in physicians.[2]

Several hundred physicians were offered an eight-week program built around mindfulness training, with close to a year of follow up. Doctors reported an increased sense of well-being, less stress, and "increased attitudes associated with patient-centered care." They reported improved mood, along with decreased tension, anger, and fatigue.

Or course, physicians have no exclusivity on burnout. Teachers, construction workers, psychologists, firefighters—we all are at risk. Any program that reduces burnout and increases empathy benefits any vocation including, without a doubt, parenting.

Other studies have suggested that mindfulness may proactively shield people from emotional stress. In February 2010, Dr. Amishi Jha at the University of Pennsylvania published a study titled "Examining the Protective Effects of Mindfulness Training on Working Memory and Emotional Experiences." With the cooperation of the military, marines waiting for deployment completed an eight-week mindfulness program.[3]

It's hard to imagine the stress felt by soldiers waiting to leave for battle. Dr. Jha found that after training in mindfulness there were less negative feelings reported by soldiers. They were better able to manage their fear. This change could have represented a blunting of overall emotion, or a shutting down of feeling, a common way humans manage when overwhelmed. Instead, Dr. Jha found something much more encouraging: For people practicing mindfulness in the face of a huge life stress, unpleasant events weren't as traumatizing as they could have been, and the soldiers also reported that enjoyable experiences were still as enjoyable as ever.

The lead up to deployment typically affects a soldier's working memory, the place in our minds where we hold onto and manipulate information as it is encountered. Under stress these core cognitive skills, vital for problem solving and learning, usually degenerate. After mindfulness training, those who consistently practiced their exercises were protected against this loss of mental ability. Mindfulness appeared to shield them from the mental effects of stress.

⚬≫⚬

Mindfulness programs improve executive function and attention skills and foster emotional regulation. Clinical studies, research on attention, and examination of brain functioning after meditation all suggest profound benefits. Most studies are not of monks or people who meditate extraordinary amounts of time. They instead look at people who take a six- or eight-week class, or meditate less than half an hour daily for a stretch of time.

One of the initial studies completed by Dr. Kabat Zinn involved patients with psoriasis. Psoriasis is a chronic skin condition that causes dry plaques to form on various areas of the body. In rare cases, it can cover people from nearly head to toe.

One intervention uniformly works in these extreme situations. Intense ultraviolet light treatments resolve an outbreak of psoriasis every time. However, the number of treatments required varies greatly among patients, requiring several weekly visits over a series of months. This chronic exposure to ultraviolet light puts people at risk for skin cancer, so limiting the number of treatments is ideal.

In an early study of mindfulness-based stress reduction, some patients with psoriasis were given guided meditation tapes during their light treatments. Another group sat through the treatment as usual. At the conclusion of the study, the meditation group had required 30 percent fewer light treatments.[4]

Mindfulness interventions have since been shown to reduce symptoms related to chronic pain, insomnia, rheumatoid arthritis, and a host of other conditions. For cancer patients, mindfulness does not cure their disease, but it can change how they perceive their quality of life. People completing mindfulness classes demonstrate a stronger immune response. In another study, people who spent eight weeks practicing mindfulness had a more robust, protective response to getting a flu vaccine than people who got the same shot but didn't take the course.[5]

Remarkably, a small 2009 study of patients with HIV showed similar results. The health of patients with HIV depends on the maintenance of white blood cell counts, since white blood cells fight infection. Cell counts remained constant in the group taking an MBSR class, and fell at a typical rate for another group of patients who attended a one-day general stress reduction seminar.[6]

Reading all of this, you may wonder if mindfulness sounds too good to be true. While studies are ongoing, month by month more research is published regarding both new and potential ways mindfulness can help us enhance our lives. But the greater answer may simply be this: The effect of mindfulness on well-being and chronic stress may alter the course of almost any psychological or physical condition.

∽∾

Research integrating mindfulness and the field of psychology has exploded over the last decade as well. Specific applications have been developed for conditions as diverse as depression, borderline personality disorder, and insomnia. Beyond benefiting individual conditions, a theme emerges throughout these papers. People who practice mindfulness report an enhanced sense of overall well-being.

Psychologists in England have developed a program called mindfulness-based cognitive therapy for depression (MBCT). This program integrates traditional cognitive therapy techniques with mindfulness training. One of the concepts introduced through MBCT is that our moods often fluctuate, but how we respond varies from person to person. If we have a tendency for depression, as our mood drops we may rapidly fall into ruminative thoughts: *Oh no, here I go again. I can't handle it. I'm going to be miserable.*

When you break the mental cycle you often stop the rumination, reminding yourself, perhaps, that "thoughts are just thoughts." Your mood may be low, but you pull back from the precipice and avoid a full episode of depression.

The actual MBCT program is much more intricate. It involves intensive patient education and other therapeutic techniques. Regardless, the program has been so successful that it is recommended for depression by England's national health program. In adults with a history of chronic depression, the rate of relapse dropped from 66 percent to 37 percent after completing the MBCT program.[7]

Many studies demonstrate benefits for anxiety—and not only for clinical anxiety disorders, but for the day-to-day stress that comes and goes for all of us. College students who completed a *one-week* intervention with meditation training offered for twenty minutes a day reported feeling happier and less anxious while performing a challenging task and had lower blood levels of cortisol, a stress hormone.[8] Another study showed increased pain tolerance and decreased anxiety in college students after one hour of mindfulness training divided over three days.[9]

The skill of noticing and labeling inner emotional states may be beneficial for stress all on its own. A UCLA study showed that the simple act of verbalizing an internal feeling minimized its emotional impact. Researchers used MRIs to document that once negative emotions were expressed and described, stress induced by those emotions seemed to shut off in the brain.[10]

Studies have looked at what happens in family relationships when parents complete a mindfulness program. Parents of children with developmental disabilities and autism completed classes and reported less parenting stress, increased social interaction with their children, and more comfort with their parenting abilities. Children with intense behavioral problems showed improved behavior after their parents completed the program.[11] Another pilot study conducted in 2009 examined parent-child pairs where the children had ADHD. Children's compliance improved when their parents completed mindfulness training. Compliance improved even further when the kids completed a similar program, modified for their age.[12]

Brain Benefits

Exactly how flexible our minds are in training attention remains to be seen. But we know the basics—attention is a fundamentally trainable skill. A motivated adult, such as anyone practicing mindfulness, can improve attention to some degree much like they would build muscles through weight lifting. Can we document physical changes that parallel these clinical benefits?

On a simple level, when people report feelings of optimism and well-being, neurons in the left frontal lobes are found to be firing more than those in the right. When the ratio shifts, people are more likely to be sad, or feel pessimistic. After two months of beginning meditation and mindfulness instruction, people in one study not only said they felt better, but electrical activity in the brain showed a shift to the left.[13] Other brain scan studies have demonstrated similar benefits, such as increased synchronization in electrical firings in the brain, which also correlates with feelings of well-being.

A study at Harvard University observed physical development in the brains of people who meditate. Dr. Sara Lazar measured the thickness of the brain's outer layers—the grey matter—over the frontal cortex in two groups of people. The outer cortex thins during adulthood, and cortical thinning of this kind correlates with memory loss and the onset of conditions such as Alzheimer's disease. The control group, who had never meditated, showed typical thinning over time. The group of mediators? There was no thinning at all. Dr. Lazar also noted thickening in the area of the brain called the insula, which is involved in emotional regulation.[14]

Expectations and Stress

On the one hand, stressful, unpleasant events are inevitable in life, which is why mindfulness does not promise stress elimination. On the other hand, the actual experience of stress frequently stems from our thoughts—a fearful image triggers a concrete chemical chain in our body. This frightening thought is not the same as actual danger, so not everything that induces stress is inherently unsafe. While we cannot change the fact that stress will find us, we can begin to change how we respond.

Continuing the discussion of stress from chapter four, the cascade of physical and emotional stress started by the amygdala works like an on-and-off switch, without much room for nuance. I'm afraid, I'm not afraid. I'm safe, I'm not safe. Run. Don't run. Thousands of years ago, this type of reaction was, most likely, quite useful. Under threat from animals, starvation, or other humans, we developed a complex series of reactions to survive. The amygdala fired and our adrenaline kicked in, blood flow shifted from our digestive system to our muscles. We coiled to react, to protect ourselves from danger.

The amygdala does not discriminate. Fear is fear. Thoughts enter our minds—I have too much to do today, I have to get to the doctor by two and pick up the dry cleaning and something for dinner and my back is sore and and and... and that's it, the amygdala fires and we feel wound up and stressed.

Very often, there is no real risk to our well-being. The to-do list will get done—or it won't. Through mindfulness we begin to note the process—the tendency to escalate from an idle thought to a physical surge of hormones and reactions. If we catch ourselves before reacting, we can stop. That's only a thought. I'm busy today—that's all. And then return to the breath one more time.

⁓∞⁓

Humans are talented at perpetuating our own stress. We're wired to protect ourselves, but often go overboard. Rattled by something, we immediately push back or run away. Our thoughts snake into the past, tie our present situation to a string of experiences that are long gone. Or they unravel into the future, and we become agitated and then remain on guard because of a cascade of worry.

Afraid of what we imagine, we might fall back on denial, twisting the facts. They're just a kid. That's how I was. Their teacher is too hard on them. Or we may paint pictures of the future, and create expectations that cannot be met—I'm starting to meditate and by next month I'll be completely without stress and my child will behave better and life will be perfect. These strings of thought maintain our unrest.

Emotions trigger their own stress cycles. I'm feeling down today. I'm on edge, there must be a reason, there must be something I can fix. And then, your problem-solving mind fires up and looks for a solution. Your mind ratchets up, adrenaline flows, and all the related defensive processes continue.

The physical state of our body perpetuates stress. We may tense our muscles or become fidgety at first, but then our minds notice our body's responses. Our shoulders are hunched, or our head feels off, or we're scowling…and we assume we are on edge for a reason. Off we go into thought and problem solving again, and the amygdala continues to fire.

Sleep deprivation enables stress. Exercise, for most people, decreases it, when we find the time. Caffeine—as much as many of us enjoy it—often pushes our stress level higher. What we consume and the life style choices we make in general all influence how at ease we will feel day to day. In all these different ways stress fuels itself, until we notice the pattern, and take a new direction.

And of course, we also often grab onto pictures we have of how life *should* be. You're in New York, and decide to head to the Bronx Zoo. They have this great new exhibit that has a white alligator, and everyone in the family seems excited. You herd your son out the door, and your blood pressure is rising because the zoo closes at four thirty in the winter, and the day is slipping away.

You arrive at the zoo. It's two, he's hungry, you pause for a snack, and he becomes completely engaged in relishing his hot chocolate. And then wants to ride the carousel. And meanwhile, you're 90 percent focused on getting to see any actual animal—much less the alligator—before closing.

There you are. You're on vacation and with him at the zoo. But you have this picture—we need to see an animal, and you wanted to show him the alligator. Actually, you wanted to see the alligator yourself. You're nudging him to move, calculating in your head how many more minutes until it's too late, how long a walk is it from here to there. And you're stressed—because your picture of the day, apparently, is quite different from his. He's having a blast. And you, most certainly, are not.

Respond, Not React

Paying attention to how we experience our daily lives lays the foundation for change. We become familiar with the feelings, thoughts, emotions, and details of our interactions with the world around us. Breaking our self-perpetuating cycles of reactivity begins with this level of awareness. We practice patience, the ability to pause and return to the moment and to respond with equanimity to challenges.

Not every thought or emotion merits an action—although they often feel like they do. So often, emotions are passing states of mind, either entirely random or momentarily triggered. Your mood crashes because you are exhausted. Unconsciously you might start to search for why you feel down—it must be because of my daughter, when will she get her act together?

But if we're uncomfortable because of a state of mind, we cannot always fix that. Sometimes we start looking outside of ourselves and place blame. I must feel bad for a reason. There is a false assumption that every internal state—"I feel rotten"—has a distinct, correctible cause. In fact, our mood may have shifted all on its own, or maybe we're just overtired or drank too much coffee.

As well, the world is never perfectly stable and safe and unchanging for any length of time. We're going to feel a little unsettled at some point. It's inevitable—and it is an inner experience that does not necessarily resolve just because we reach out and do something to it, for it, or about it. Shutting down the stress cycle may start with a shift of perspective, accepting that the discomfort around a situation is nothing more than discomfort.

When feeling off balance, we may shut down, actively ignore problems, or strike back at the world around us. I'm stuck. I'm scared. Leave me alone. We feel off, so we get angry or anxious or become enervated or obsessively focus on problems. And then we try to do something to alter the world around us, to avoid that feeling of uncertainty. We overplan, or ruminate, or go for a drink, or overeat.

Children are particularly skilled at triggering the unsettling sensation that life is not fully in our control. We have these great ideas about how to be a parent, what to say in some particular circumstance, or how a child should live their life. And then somewhere in early childhood they develop their own personality and will. We pictured long hikes in the woods, they want only to play baseball and hockey. We think that they'd be a brilliant engineer, and they want to major in English.

And day to day, it turns out we cannot affect every aspect of our child's behavior. We want a guarantee a situation will turn out as we pictured, and our child leads us down a different path. We're sitting at a wedding and we'd really like them to remain in their seat and stop making noise, and, in spite of all our best efforts, they simply will not. We're finally at the head of the line at the grocery store and out of nowhere, there's a tantrum.

The sensation of instability is magnified when caring for some-one with ADHD. Right now, today, your child has her own strengths, and perhaps a long list of ADHD-related difficulties. You're doing a lot to make changes. There may have been improvements but issues persist. You may have had a nagging sense of fear, for months or years, a wish that you could know for sure that everything is going to work out as you hope. Instead of reacting to the feeling or shutting down, you can build an attitude of, okay, I feel unsure, take a breath, it's normal to feel this way.

One of the first concepts that connects for many people tak-ing a stress reduction class is "responding, not reacting." Instead of saying or doing something reflexively, we build an ability to stop a moment, gather ourselves, and choose what comes next. But to know when to pause—when to make sure we're not being reac-tive—we have to be aware of our unconscious habits in the first place.

Sitting here reading this book or meditating or having dinner, that sense of unbalance may be hanging around you. Acting on it—by obses-sively problem solving or drinking or exercising or reading or yelling or anything else—may temporarily distract you from the discomfort. Another perspective is to notice it, and what it feels like. Recognize, this is how I am when I'm off balance—and I don't need to act at all until I'm ready.

⁓⊗⁓

There is a common assumption that if we wrestle with a problem long enough, we will find a definite resolution. This makes sense for some concrete issues, situations where a particular action will lead to a likely conclusion. But for emotional experiences, there can be a backward logic to it. You might be thinking, if only I struggle with this complex series of completely illogical thoughts and emotions long enough, I'll be at peace.

In reality, the opposite may be true. When we start at a place of peace, the complicated thoughts and emotions grab us less, become less intense, and may even resolve themselves. Are you stressed and ruminating because some problem has taken over your mind, or has some problem taken over your mind because you are stressed? We may assume we'll be happy as soon as we stop ruminating. More likely, though, if we can find a way to feel less stressed, then we'll stop ruminating.

Again, nothing about the practice of mindfulness means that life will never be stressful, or make us angry, or be painful, and trying to notice your responses in various stressful situations without self-judgment can be challenging. When your child decides to toss a milkshake across a restaurant, it doesn't mean that you have "failed" at meditation when you get angry. It's never a failure to get flustered or upset. Like stress, those moments are inevitable, and all that we control is how we respond to them.

THE BODY SCAN

The body scan is another method you can use to break the stress cycle. In the body scan, you pay attention to sensations in your body, as always without forcing anything in particular to happen along the way. Many people find this exercise relaxing, but you might feel restless or sleepy or anything else. Whatever your experience, you are still cultivating mindfulness through the practice of paying attention.

You can choose any comfortable, stable place to practice the body scan, a chair, or your bed, or using cushions or mats on the floor. Lying or sitting in a comfortable position, start by bringing your attention to your breath. Take a few gentle breaths, and notice the rising and falling of your stomach. Wherever you find it easy, let go of tension you feel in your body. If lying down, let your arms and legs fall gently to the side, and if sitting, let your hands rest easily on your thighs or together in your lap.

If you prefer to do the body scan lying down, choose a time of day where you aren't overly tired. Keep your eyes open instead of closed if you find it helpful in staying awake. You can even hold your hands gently together in the air over your midsection; you'll notice them moving if you start to drift off.

The body scan is a useful relaxation tool for some. It may even help you unwind for sleep—a slightly different use than as an alert, focused meditation. If you find it useful for sleep, enjoy it and maybe complete a different meditation some other time during the day.

Bring your attention first to your feet, either one or both. Try to notice any sensations you feel, like warmth or cold, dampness or dryness. You might notice nothing at all, and that's normal too. And then slowly, pausing along the way, move your attention from your feet up along your body to your head. Spend several minutes paying attention to each area of your body, step by step from your lower legs to your knees to your hips, and then upward. Pace yourself, continuing to relax whatever tension you can let go of easily, but not trying to force yourself to feel anything.

If there is discomfort anywhere along the way, notice that. If you're able to maintain your attention on this area, observe the sensations for a little while—they likely wax and wane, changing their quality over time. If the feeling is too intense, shift your attention away to another area of your body, or to the breath. And at any point if you need to move then pause a moment and, with intention, choose the moment that you shift. Make whatever adjustments you need, whenever you need them.

The body scan also helps you become aware of subtle sensations in your body related to feelings, thoughts, and emotions. Once in a while you may begin to notice your body reacting before your mind takes over—*my shoulders are tight, my jaw is tense.* And when in meditation, or in life, you find your mind swept away in thought or emotion, you can often ground yourself by returning to the sensations in the body—feeling yourself sitting in a chair or the wind in your face. You may pull a discursive mind out of its ruts for a moment, letting thoughts settle and emotions calm.

Take Time for Yourself

Our hectic lives as parents often seem written in stone. *I can't catch up. I have no time for myself, and probably never will. From when I wake to when I sleep, I'm busy, I have things to do. I cannot possibly find fifteen minutes to meditate.*

We're overscheduled. We have loads of responsibilities and sprawling to-do lists. All true. But is every moment truly spoken for, every day? If someone offered you one thousand dollars for each time you sat in meditation, would you find a way to make it happen?

If you've committed to some time for yourself, protect it and schedule it. Track several days on a calendar if needed. How much time do you take answering e-mail? Surfing the Internet? Watching television?

How much time do you play with your child, or talk to your spouse? Could the household chores be juggled? Could you wake up fifteen minutes earlier?

There is no one way to start—chose a plan and stick to it as best you can. And when you stop practicing for a stretch, treat yourself as you would during meditation. Notice you've gotten off track, pause, and recommit to the lifestyle you've chosen.

THE MYTH OF MULTI-TASKING

Multitasking turns out to be an ineffective way of living. We might, in any moment, feel pulled by four or five pressing things we have to do, and problems we have to solve. It often feels most efficient to do them all simultaneously. Or we may feel that we have no choice but to attack everything at once.

But our minds can only pay attention to one object at a time. When we juggle ideas, we're not processing several in parallel—we're rapidly moving back and forth between them, and not paying full attention to anything. In reality, multi-tasking increases the time any individual task takes, and makes it more likely we'll make mistakes along the way.

By building the skill of attention management, it becomes easier to place your attention where you want. Each perceived problem or item on your to-do list still grabs at you, but you can focus on each activity in full, moving others to the side. You can reach a point of resolution, or choose a moment to pause, and then shift to the next point. Both your overall efficiency and effectiveness will improve.

The traditional mindfulness-based stress reduction program recommends meditating forty-five minutes a day. It is a commitment to radical change, a shift in how you experience your daily life. If you can do that, great, the investment will pay off—but that's not the only way to start.

Commit to ten minutes in the car after parking on the way into the office, and ten minutes before leaving for home. Fifteen minutes at the end of lunch hour. Fifteen *breaths*, once an hour through the day—one minute an hour, as a starting point, to settle yourself. Everything is completely falling apart around me and I'm going to be the one to pause, for these few moments, before moving forward.

⚬◇⚬

Ian, a participant in a mindfulness class I was leading, had two kids with ADHD and worked at a mile-a-minute commodities firm. He spent every minute in the office connected to his cell phone, e-mail, and computer. After a few weeks of class, he commented about watching the smokers in his office building.

Smoking had been banned indoors. Many times a day, the smokers would gather, walk to the elevator, wait patiently, and ride down to the ground floor. Walk outside. Smoke a cigarette. Stroll back in the elevator. Ride upstairs. Jump back into the hectic financial mix. And no one thought twice about the breaks they had taken.

After two weeks of struggling to find meditation time, Ian actually notices the smokers in action. They're leaving their desks, over and over again. Their world isn't ending. They still have their jobs. Why can't I just shut my door for two minutes and breathe?

So he did.

⚬◇⚬

While mindfulness can develop without meditation, meditation is a proven and profoundly helpful tool. As we train our attention, we become more aware of how we think and where our mind runs throughout the day. We break the cycle of autopilot, time spent moving through life without paying attention, and without making conscious and intentional choices about what we say or do. We use focused attention to become more aware of the unconscious perceptions and experiences that influence our behavior. We pay more attention to our mental habits, and we develop the ability to pause, reflect, and make skillful new choices. Coupled with a thorough understanding of ADHD, managing your own stress and cultivating openness to new ways of handling challenges lays the groundwork for transforming your family's life with ADHD.

CHAPTER 6

Taking Care of Yourself: Mindfulness in Action

Practicing mindfulness, we try to get out of "autopilot"—mindlessly running around lost in thought, reacting to situations without foresight. In bringing our attention to our moment-to-moment experience, we'll still find some parts of life pleasant and others unpleasant. We also build the skill of noticing and labeling the sensations we experience, our thoughts and our emotions—an essential component of mental health. And as we become familiar with our habits, we often recognize what we have been doing unconsciously, and then have the option of choosing a new path.

༺∽༻

You might wonder, what does following my breath or noticing that my feet feel warm have to do with my child's ADHD? It's a fair question and the answer is, you have to start somewhere. You want to break lifelong habits and develop new coping tools, but you cannot begin in the midst of a behavioral crisis. That's why most of the mindfulness exercises offered throughout this book examine far less emotionally charged aspects of life than your interactions with your child. As you get more practiced, you'll expand toward more challenging moments and even then, the opportunity to return to your breath will be available as a calming and less daunting focus for your mind.

This chapter offers an overview of mindfulness techniques—your first steps toward a new way of living your life and managing your child's ADHD. Interspersed throughout are exercises you can try at your own pace and return to over time. The chapter ends with a six-week program outline for those who would like to work with these tools in a more structured fashion.

Stepping into Life

There I was in this store and my two boys were running around, I didn't know exactly where. I was looking for new jackets for them. I'd never get it done if I chased them around. And then the store manager came up and said to me, "Your kids are running up and down stairs with a $400 fishing pole," and without thinking I said, "Why were they able to get their hands on a $400 fishing pole?" He looked kind of stunned, and I felt like I'd won. And then I looked around the store. Several people had heard, and two had their kids right with them. All of sudden I realized, how come I was the only one whose kids were out of control? It was the first moment I recognized, something has to change.

⸎

Without effort, we live out our lives barely paying attention to what is going on around us. We spend so much of our time not quite here. We carve out a little time to relax and go for a run, and then instead of taking the time to recharge we spend the time mentally rehashing our financial situation. Reading a book with our child at bedtime, we dwell on a problem at work. Wherever we are in life, our minds are often off somewhere else, not fully involved with the world around us.

When we live on autopilot, something rattles us and we stay lost in thought. We may dwell or ruminate afterward—*I can't believe they said that. I should have kept my mouth shut. Next time what I'm going to say is*...and through all that extra thought, we're not paying attention to our lives as they are happening.

We often lose out on brief moments of peace. Frustrated that the morning unraveled, we fail to take advantage of ten minutes respite as our children board the bus. Our bodies and minds remain in stress mode. We're ready for action, agitated, and formulating what we'll say next time around. But we're actually in a quiet, warm house drinking our morning coffee.

We might yell when our children misbehave because we always have yelled, and it gets them in line. And our children have learned their own habits, their own autopilot. They've learned they don't have to listen until we start yelling. Everything until then is play time. Since anything we do repetitively becomes hardwired, these well-worn paths exist in our brains. A pattern we fall back on becomes that much easier to trigger the next time around, regardless of whether it is particularly skillful, or what we'd recommend for a friend in the same situation.

We all have our ways of responding when challenged. Tripping on the way to the podium, one speaker might think, *What a klutz I am.* Another might think, *How embarrassing, they're all laughing at me.* Another might lash out, *Who left their bag in the aisle? You nearly killed me.*

We can't expect to, and nor should we want to, strip ourselves of every habit. Each response has a time and a place. Being obsessive about cleanliness and detail is imperative for a surgeon in the operating room. Maintaining that same standard with your family kitchen? Perhaps a cause of stress. What is skillful and brilliant in one situation may not apply in another.

No habits are inherently better than any others. At some time in life, you'll want to stand up to the world. At some point, you'll want to take stock of yourself and withdraw. There's a time to yell, to react with fear, to hyperfocus on a crisis until it is solved. Awareness of our habits allows us to pick and choose which we give weight to; our lives do not need to be dominated by them. There's nothing right or wrong about most habits, but there's no need to let them run your life.

Direct Your Attention

Mindfulness, on one level, is a simple tool. Any time during the day you can pause, take a few breaths, and settle yourself. Almost any activity can be done meditatively—why *not* focus on our families while we're with them? When it's time to work, work, and if you need to fix the dishwasher, go fix it. At its most basic, the practice is focusing our attention away from mental distractions, back to our lives as they happen. Easy to say, challenging to live.

Meditation may conjure up images of beatific individuals smiling blissfully, eyes closed, off lost in the woods. But that type of escape isn't the point. Mindfulness meditation isn't about running away, or self-analysis. It's about the opposite—stripping away whatever barriers keep us outside of our daily lives.

Relaxation is not even a goal in and of itself; instead, we strive for a sense of balance. If we become too relaxed, we fall asleep, or in certain situations might find ourselves defenseless. Nor do we want to be too tense, battling our minds to focus without a break. We seek instead a stability between alertness and calm.

While there is a larger goal of becoming more familiar with our experience and habits, practicing mindfulness is not meant to be therapy. In therapy, people explore the cause and effect of their emotions and behaviors, and focus on problem solving. Through mindfulness meditation, we're not trying to analyze our mental states or patterns of thought. We're trying to become familiar with them. We cannot compel ourselves to a particular state of relaxation or wisdom or happiness. We're slowing down and watching, developing an unbiased, awareness of our lives that builds a sense of steadfastness and composure. Skillful choices and insights often follow.

We also cultivate an attitude during the experience of meditation. When the mind wanders we try to return to the breath without frustration or self-flagellation. So you became distracted? Great job, you noticed that and focused yourself again. That's the practice; however many hundreds of times you become distracted, striving to come back with a measure of compassion.

Even on days when meditation is immensely challenging—our minds on fire with excitement or anxiety, happiness or grief—doing our best to return to our actual experience is still practicing. We observe, watching things change and letting things be for a few minutes. We pause and let the dust settle, hoping to see our lives with clarity.

Practicing the release of any compulsion to be doing something every moment of our lives, fixing and solving and planning all the time, we protect some time and space to quiet down. Not everything in life can be controlled, and there can be strength in not doing anything.

You can practice mindfulness through any moment in daily life, even mundane chores. You can wash the dishes while annoyed and pressured because you want to be doing something else, but if the dishes need to be done anyway, why not elect to do them without adding on layers of stress? Pay attention to the details, the warm water and sounds of the plates moving, and notice when your thoughts are off elsewhere. You cannot force any activity to become enjoyable, but you can focus away from mental distractions, back to the moment at hand.

Or not. With practice, you step out of autopilot and decide when to pay attention. You might make a conscious choice to avoid thinking of some other chore—someone has to clean up after the dog in the backyard. That's going to be a nasty experience, as it was the last dozen times. So instead of focusing your full attention on the unpleasantness, focus on something else, like your next vacation.

Experience the Moment

Practicing mindfulness is not only about how we approach challenging experiences. With almost anything we do in life we add layers, some of which may complicate even a straightforward, pleasurable moment. Finding a break, we take a walk and feel guilty for not working, or for leaving our children with a babysitter, or for simply getting lost in daydreaming. Attending a concert we might find ourselves thinking *this is great, I can't wait to tell my wife about it, I need to remember exactly what he played, let's see, first he played*... and now we're not paying full attention to the music.

When you're with your children, you can focus on playing with them. You can be mindful about driving—not meditating, but paying full attention to driving and nothing else. When eating, just eat. You don't have to shovel in food, barely tasting it along the way. Pause between bites. Enjoy yourself. Slow down and notice, in a relaxed, unstilted way, the experience of eating.

As an exercise, try eating a piece of fruit as if it was the first time you ever encountered it. Imagine you're deciding if it is edible, if it is safe to eat, or what it might taste like. Don't force anything to happen. Explore, noticing each of your five senses—vision, then touch, then smell; listen to any sounds the fruit makes, moving it around in your hand.

Before placing it in your mouth, pause. Notice any sensations in your mouth or body as you hold still. Choose the moment you move your hand, paying attention to your muscles along the way. Notice any urge to rush, to move quicker, to eat, or to quit. And then again, with intention, decide when to chew, paying attention to taste, and then swallow.

As soon as you start, your mind likely kicks in. You might feel awkward and think, *this exercise is lame.* Or you might enjoy it, and think, *this tastes good, what a great way to celebrate food.* Both are normal responses. For almost any experience in life, our mind reacts with this instant classification into good, bad, or neither.

Most of us recognize that when eating slower we eat healthier and enjoy our food more. Instead of eating raisins by the handful, we can choose to taste them, yet few of us eat with such care day to day. Once a day, or once a week, pay attention to nothing but the food in front of you as you eat. It can be a three-course event at an upscale restaurant, or a snack on a crowded subway car. Wherever you are, this eating meditation is available, helping you focus out of your thoughts onto the simple act of eating.

Good Judgment

I'm hardly even telling anyone we started medication. There's all this chatter when people do. They don't even think about what's it's been like for us, or for our son Alan. My husband isn't constantly correcting him anymore. They sit and play a whole game together. Alan has this chart at school, red lights for bad behavior, green for good. All of a sudden he's getting green every day. He's talking about it all the time. He's playing longer with kids. And still, there's so much judgment about using medication, like we couldn't deal, or we're trying some kind of band-aid.

⌒∞⌒

Judgment is so much a part of life when you have a child with ADHD. Someone feels that your child is not acting right, that his behavior is inappropriate and you are responsible. A magazine article or a relative suggests that ADHD comes from parenting, and you feel the statement is directed entirely at you. You choose medication and feel judgment from people who disagree. You choose not to use medication, and someone criticizes your choice.

Returning to the basic definition, mindfulness is often defined as a being fully aware of what is happening in the present moment *without judgment*. Without judgment means without the reflexive, often reactive categorization of our lives into good, bad, and neutral; this last group we often dismiss as not worth a moment's thought. Being nonjudgmental does not mean meekly accepting the status quo. When something needs addressing, we still do what we need to protect ourselves and make hard choices to solve problems.

There is a difference between idling in traffic trying to figure out another driving route, and sitting in traffic stewing about being late for an appointment. Anger arises—*there shouldn't be traffic right now, I shouldn't have driven this way*—but there is, and you did. There's nothing else to be done. All that angst and frustration inside, and the traffic outside hasn't budged.

We can strive to tell the difference between clear thoughts—*I need to find another way to work; I need to call ahead and let people know I'll be late*—and judgment—*why didn't I leave earlier, why can't they just get this traffic jam cleared, they must be completely incompetent.* Practically, you might instead resolve, once you calmed down, not to follow the same route again.

Mindfulness therefore requires separating the terms "judgment" and "discernment." Judgment mindlessly categorizes experience and often leads us to wrestle with what is not in our control. Discernment is recognizing what we can and should change, and what we cannot, much like the traditional serenity prayer: To accept what we cannot change, to change what we must, and to find the wisdom to tell the difference.

∾⟨∾

There are certainly moments in life that demand instant action based on the quick assessment of a situation. Years ago on a hike in Costa Rica I was stepping over a log when my body froze in midstride. Looking down, I saw a poisonous snake coiled in the shadows. My reflexes were faster than my conscious mind. I'd stopped before I could have said why and saved myself, an ability I prefer to keep honed and at the ready.

Long ago on the path of evolution, our judgments and reactions expanded far beyond their practical usefulness. Intense fear or stress often focuses our thoughts for a period of time. We lose all awareness of the greater world. This is a perfectly useful response as long as the acute danger lasts, but not so much when we return to daily life. But for most of us life isn't a matter of moment-to-moment survival anymore.

Judgment has its uses. You'll still have likes and dislikes, and unpleasant experiences are still unpleasant, even after practicing mindfulness. "No way, I'm leaving" may be a skilled response when you notice someone lurking as you enter a dark alley. But it may be a less-than-useful voice of fear that you hear when walking into a job interview. In the second case, you might notice your reaction, pause, take a few breaths, and open the door.

There's never a goal of getting rid of thoughts, either. Thoughts are going to come and go. We can note them, without becoming completely enmeshed. *My child needs to do better in school? Great, let's make a plan tonight. Right now, I'm playing baseball with him. Everything else going on in my mind is judgment, thought, emotion.*

❧

Judgment is often triggered by thoughts and social interactions more than any concrete, acute danger. A simple, common belief—my kids *should* act differently—escalates our stress level. It is a judgment of the situation—life *should* be different. But life can never be different than it *is* as we're living through any particular moment.

We recoil—my child should not have ADHD. Or maybe we think, it is not right that I feel overwhelmed, other people have it worse than I do. But your child does have ADHD. And you really are overwhelmed, even though you know other people face greater challenges.

We often compare our lives to some standard or expectation—this is not what I pictured. And then we reactively get angry or sad or anxious. But things are as they are, and there's typically nothing we can do it about it in this exact moment. This isn't meant in any stilted way. It's simple truth. The only thing we can affect in life is whatever we decide to do next.

SELF DOUBT, MOVE OUT

"Ordinarily, we spend all our time comparing and discriminating between this and that, always looking around for something good to happen to us. And because of that we become restless and anxious about everything. As long as we are able to imagine something better than what we have or who we are, it follows naturally that there could also be something worse. We are constantly pursued by misgivings that something bad will happen. In other words, as long as we live by distinguishing between the better way and the worse way, we can never find absolute peace that whatever happens is all right."[1]

We often hold ourselves to different standards than we hold the rest of the world. We love our children unconditionally, even when we are frustrated or angry. When they mess up, we try to give them the benefit of the doubt: *You were trying your hardest. You made a mistake and I still love you. You'll do better next time.*

But with ourselves, our standards can be brutal. We strive to be perfect, and when we mess up we're harsh. There even may be a subtle sense that someone else—a parent, or a spouse, or a social group—is watching, judging our actions moment to moment.

We're often overly influenced by this perfectionism and insecurity. There's a "negativity bias" inherent in human nature, a tendency to focus on things we perceive as bad. These biases potentially cause us to feel insecure or inadequate in aspects of our lives, and then we may make decisions that protect our ego, or insulate ourselves from distress. When finding some sense of acceptance of ourselves as we are right now, we begin to make settled choices about our lives.

We label and judge everything we experience, from the moment we wake until the moment we fall asleep again: *That was a good thought. That made me angry. That person looks like someone I'd like to meet. That person looks surly and unpleasant. I shouldn't judge people so quickly.*

Practice noticing this voice of judgment through the day. When you are meditating, note it and come back to your breath again, or sensations in your body, or whatever you've chosen. If you are hanging out with your children, come back to your children. Wherever you are, develop an awareness of thoughts you have that include *would, should,* or *could.* They often suggest judgment.

Practice separating your own clear-sighted perceptions from these random judgments created by the reactive mind. Notice the voice of judgment as nothing more than another thought. Letting it go, focus your attention wherever else you choose instead.

As we sit and slow down and start to become familiar with how we think, judgment crops up again and again. Instead of accepting it as reality, we can notice it as nothing more than another thought. Pay attention to the random voices that heckle and demean you through the day. If someone else said them—if a relative gave you an ear piece and said "I'm going to give you a little helpful advice for the rest of your life"—what would you do? Odds are you'd find a way to get rid of the ear piece.[2]

Practice Pausing

We notice a change in our reactions and in the kids, too. After I meditate I can carry it over to our lives and have even talked to the girls about it. I'm calmer. I don't shout as much. My kids have been taking breaths when upset, counting to ten. They're sticking out a disagreement without resorting to yelling. All good stuff.

❦

Once we recognize judgment—there's that voice again—then what do we do? Left unchecked, our emotional reactivity takes over our conscious minds. A sensation appears. Immediately, liking or disliking follows. This feels good or bad, this is how it should or shouldn't be. These reactions lead to other thoughts, reactions, and then snap decisions. We add layers upon layers to moments that were complicated enough to start.

Instead of reacting, falling back on what is mindlessly familiar, pause. Notice what you are feeling physically or emotionally. Can you begin to detect when you are starting to react, before you say or do anything? Where have your thoughts gone? What emotions are rising? Is your stomach twisted in a knot? Is your face tight? Is someone actually in danger, or is a chronic problem rearing its head again? Take a breath, reflect, and, with intention, choose what to say or do next.

No one is asking you to shut off your sense of right and wrong. Stuff happens that is fairly disagreeable in life—sometimes a lot of it. But more often than not, snap judgments and reactions limit us. A battle begins when your child doesn't want to come inside from playing. The reactions start, *This again, why can't she just come in when I call?*

So you shout out the window, *"Lisa, get in here already, I don't want to have to repeat myself!"* She ignores you, or yells something back. Day after day, you wrestle. You push her to come in sooner, she pushes back, and you both end up angry.

Stop for a moment. What's going on? Right now, today, Lisa hasn't failed to listen yet. She's happy. You were happy a moment ago. Is your anger based on anything that happened today, or is it fueled by the past? You're starting to fall into autopilot. This is what I say, this is how I feel, this is what she says, this is how she feels.

Things Change

When I was younger, I experienced intense stage fright. I'd even freeze up playing charades with a close group of friends. It didn't affect my life much; I was comfortable telling people that I wouldn't get on stage. That's all. It's not for me.

Someone would ask me to give a lecture or play a game, and my brain would leap into action. *Absolutely no way. I hate it. I'd embarrass myself. Impossible.* A line of excuses would form a traffic jam in my mind.

I assumed this trait was fixed, like my height. Then my life changed. I found a career I enjoy, I got married, I began meditating, I grew up. Whatever it was—some piece of those, or none of them—I found myself giving talks more often. Then I started getting positive feedback, being asked back to speak at the same places. One day I realized, this defining trait of mine—I hate being in the spotlight—had shifted.

There are still situations in which I'll "never" feel comfortable, like charades. And that's reactivity again. Never? Who knows? Right now, today, I'd never want to sing onstage or perform in a show (not that anyone is asking). A clenching feeling in my gut, a fearful projection even thinking about it, and yet nothing has actually happened. I'm not in danger sitting here writing about performing. Who knows what I'll think in another decade.

Even knowing that the future could be different, you still take care of yourself. Maybe down the road I'll join the circus, but for now I'm laying low. You trust your instincts, and stick to your beliefs. You make adjustments as often as necessary in order to maintain some sense of equilibrium in your life. But instead of reactively sticking to the party line—yours or anyone else's—you seek the bare facts, the reality of the broader situation.

Instead of allowing your thoughts to run ahead into fantasies of what the future might hold, pause and come back. Instead of dwelling or ruminating about what you or your child has done, notice that tendency and return. Right now, today, what would be the most skillful way for me to act, to teach, to model for my children?

Spending hours and hours in circular, emotionally driven thought leads us back to where we started. Pausing, letting go of the mental picture we painted, we try to advise ourselves like we would a close friend. Or our child.

STOP AND LET GO

In any situation, you can practice this: Listen first, breathe, and then respond. Pausing, you take a different path. You choose how to carry yourself and how to best move forward. What could you do differently? What could you show your child? If you could picture yourself in your wisest moment, what would you say or do?

An acronym used in the original MBSR program is STOP—which can serve as a reminder throughout the day:

S—Stop what you are doing
T—Take a breath (or a few)
O—Observe—what are you feeling right now, in your body and emotionally, and where are your thoughts?
P—Proceed—with intention, choose what you will say or do next

---

Building Compassion

I was putting so much pressure on myself, and my son Stephan. He has ADHD. We've tried so many different things to get him to listen. And we go to my mother-in-law's, and there's this look she gives me. It's like, without saying a word, she's staring me down. I know what she's thinking—honey, do something and get your monster under control. Or it might be in a restaurant, not that we really go anymore. Everyone is watching, and I get so angry at myself for even trying to go out for a meal. And I'm angry at Stephan. I'm doing everything I can, don't they all realize?

The list of biologically driven, ADHD-related behaviors parents blame themselves for is long. Something happens—a shove on the playground, or a social rejection—and a visceral reaction starts. I should have known this was going to happen, why didn't I do something? It's often amplified when parents do not fully comprehend or believe the biology of ADHD. Or maybe they do, but their spouse doesn't. If you cannot see ADHD as a medical condition, it's easy to assume the persistent behavior is *somebody's* fault.

My kid does not get invited to parties anymore. They don't seem to have any close friends. My spouse feels I should be doing something different with the children. My parents think I should be stricter. My friends think I should be more lenient. Their teacher thinks I am too indulgent. Their other teacher feels I should motivate them. For each of these ADHD-driven thoughts, a twinge or a deluge of self-doubt may follow. Am I doing the right thing?

You're trying to make a change, and there may be a practical step to take. But the hectoring, often abusive voice of judgment may linger. You're not good enough, you have to work harder, if only you were a better parent. If only I was a better person or you were or he was, then everything would be different. Or you think about your family. If you were a more motivated child, or if you were the kind of dad who spends more time with his kids.

We are frequently led to assume that we find happiness only when we get our act together, reach some state of perfection and answer the voices. Instead, we can notice those voices for what they are, a combination of what we actually hear from the world and our own inner commentaries. And then instead of taking it all at face value, we can train ourselves toward a more compassionate, insightful way of living.

⸙

When we are driven by an endless sense of letting ourselves down, or letting down our families, our boss, or whomever else, we exhaust our mental resources and make unskilled decisions. When we begin to notice the voice of judgment, we can begin to let it go. Thanks for the feedback, I'll take it under consideration, I did everything I could.

A subtle (or less-than-subtle) inner message criticizes every move, never satisfied. I messed up again, I should have done that better. I'll never get it right. Or it constantly compares everything as it is to what it "should" be. *Do I have the job I should, the house I should, the kids I should, or even the spouse I should?*

Perhaps one day you're hanging out on a blanket at a picnic, and someone playing Frisbee accidentally steps in your food. Looking up, you see one of your closest friends—and you smile and shrug it off. But if you look up and see someone you don't like, or don't trust at all, what then? It's the same accident, but instead you become annoyed.

Typically, we don't treat ourselves like we treat our friends. You're playing Frisbee at a company picnic and accidentally step in your boss's food. Immediately, you are flooded with a pile of thoughts, feelings, body sensations. Maybe your stomach flips, your palms sweat. You might have reflexive thoughts about yourself. *How careless. Fool. Why weren't you more careful?* All without nearly the patience or grace you would have had for your closest friend, a moment ago. Driven by these unconscious, negative judgments, where does your behavior go? What might you say or do? How clear would you be in your next choices?

Aware of their influence, you might notice when they arise—and choose not to listen. By cultivating for yourself the attitude you'd have toward a close friend, and by giving yourself a break, you may discover something new. I messed up, and I'm sorry. What is my next step?

⌒∞⌒

Observing the world with nothing but cold clarity would be exhausting. It wouldn't take us far towards happiness. While focusing attention back to our actual experience is part of the picture, equally important is building compassion—living our moment-to-moment lives without bias, and without reactive judgment of our experiences.

When we practice meditation, we cultivate this approach. I'm trying to focus on my breath, oops, I was distracted, and then without judgment (and therefore, with compassion) coming back. Even when we make a mistake we can cut ourselves some slack, make amends if we need to, and at the same time take into account our good intentions. Mindfulness training is an antidote to rumination and self-abuse.

Even when you did nothing intentionally wrong in any given situation, you may still hear voices of self-doubt. You start kicking yourself, or lamenting the state of your life, or flaring up in anger at your child or spouse. Noticing that, you can return your focus to wishing yourself well—may I find some peace, health, happiness, well-being, or whatever else you imagine.

While on some basic level each of us strives to find this ease and safety in life, the concept of building compassion isn't asking you to accept everything about yourself or anyone else as perfect. We all have things we could work on and improve, or new tools we might pick up. We still recognize when we're upset, things didn't go as we pictured, and it's painful.

Building compassion isn't asking us to accept everyone else's behavior as right. Our children don't do what we want all the time, and there are situations we will need to address. There are also going to be people we dislike, or others who may do us harm. While we continue trying, when possible, to see their perspective, we can still move them completely out of our lives, and act decisively to protect ourselves. Perhaps, though, we can disagree with someone without losing ourselves in vitriol, or questioning their basic intentions in life.

You can remind yourself that we're all trying our best—you and your child or husband or boss or anyone else. We all deserve to be at ease and find happiness. My child is being defiant again; they blew off their school work, and then lied about it. And I had to repeat myself fourteen times to get them to the bus. But behind all that misbehavior is what? A desire to be happy, nothing more.

You're still going to do what you need to get them on track—and then repeat to yourself, as often as needed, that they're only trying to find well being, like everyone else. In a charged, intense moment—how come you failed English, you told me last week you were getting a B—you can pause. Practice reminding yourself that whatever led to this moment, they don't want to fail English just as much as you don't want to see them fail.

Finding Empathy for ADHD

There may be a notion that children with ADHD should pull themselves up by the bootstraps, get their act together, and stop forgetting, or start to behave better. Maybe you blame your child on some level for his ADHD. *You know the rules. Do your work already. Stop acting like that.*

How does your child feel about it? Behind the bluster or silence, what's going on? Most of the time, they are suffering as much as you are. They have ADHD, with all the intrinsic difficulties it brings. They want to be settled and have friends and to learn like everyone else, and they want to succeed in your eyes. You may have battles and sullenness and layers of household tension, but what's your child's view of it all?

Recognizing their perspective doesn't release them from responsibility. You still need to set clear limits and enforce discipline. You still expect effort and kindness. And at the same time, you create long-term plans and anticipate problem situations and supply them the tools they need to thrive.

Even when you disagree with their choices, you may be able to recognize they are only trying to get by. You take stands while also recognizing that if your kids had the right tools, they'd probably stop whatever behavior you're trying to correct. Children with ADHD may misbehave or seem to lack motivation, but they want to be happy like everyone else.

◦◈◦

In building compassion and emotional resilience, we change our brains in subtle but meaningful ways. Instead of spending twenty minutes mentally lashing ourselves or our children for "failing" in some way, we can focus on a more compassionate perspective. I'm trying my best, you're trying your best. I'm trying to find some peace, and so are you. You notice the self-judgment without buying in. You notice when you harshly judge someone else, and take a step back from the thought.

On a medical level, focusing on compassion causes neurons to fire in particular parts of the brain that relate not only to compassion for others, but to our own sense of well-being. When compassion centers are firing, they change how we perceive the world. We become less likely to negatively interpret all the ambiguous information we encounter every day. They also affect how we choose to treat other people; one recent study showed that focusing on compassion improved people's attitudes towards strangers.[3]

As with most aspects of mindfulness, studies confirm benefits of this practice in daily life. One study exposed people to a challenging experience—public speaking, which is an almost universally successful method of inducing stress. People in the audience were trained to respond in an ambiguous way. Among the participants, people trained in practices that build self-compassion were less stressed and less likely to misinterpret the neutral feedback they were getting as negative.

Studies have shown physical shifts in the brain when people who meditate focus on feelings of compassion. They experience patterns of firing in the frontal lobes that correlate with a sense of ease. We appear able to change our long-term emotional states through mental exercises and concentration.[4]

Children learn empathy through observing their parents' actions and behaviors. They are born with their own innate tendencies and they watch and learn from adults around them. However you treat your children, your spouse, your friends, difficult people you encounter, salespeople, a panhandler, children observe, take unconscious notes, and build their own skills.

METTA: FINDING COMPASSION

A specific type of meditation called *metta* or *lovingkindness* builds this perspective of compassion. Lovingkindness is a biblical word, translated as far back as the 1500s, used to describe both God's nature and the feeling of a husband for his wife. It is also an approximate translation of a Southeast Asian word, *metta*, which describes this practice. The term *lovingkindness* itself really doesn't matter much; if it triggers you negatively, pay attention to the feeling and then substitute a word you find more comfortable.

In practicing *metta*, we start by focusing our attention on ourselves. We deserve happiness, safety, and ease as much as anyone else. When we're dragged down or overwhelmed by self-judgment, we limit our ability to empathize with others. Moving beyond these inner voices, we may find ourselves better able to see ourselves and the world with clarity. A traditional series of phrases represents these universal desires and is often paraphrased as, "May I be happy; may I be healthy; may I feel safe; may I live my life with ease." Begin this practice by focusing these wishes towards yourself, mentally repeating them at a measured pace, perhaps timed to the movement of your breath.

The exact phrases have no importance, so you can substitute whatever other words you like: May I not feel confused, may I feel at peace, may I feel balanced and wise. Find concepts that feel natural for you, whatever you most hope for yourself, choosing only three or four at most.

While practicing *metta* meditation, we focus on these phrases without forcing anything. You cannot make yourself feel loving or compassionate or peaceful or anything else. Feelings come and go. Notice whatever distractions come up and, without effort, return to the phrases as you would return your attention to your breathing.

After spending some time focusing on yourself, when you're ready, picture someone who has been only supportive to you over time—a benefactor for whom you have no conflicting emotions. Perhaps it's someone close, or a mentor, or a person outside your life who inspires you, or someone you've never met. If no person comes to mind (it's common), then stay with yourself, continuing with the same phrases for as long as you would like.

Next, without rushing, move your attention to a friend. You might picture the first person who comes to mind. You might find a friend who truly needs your support right now in some way, someone sick or struggling. Focus the same intention, with the same phrases, on your friend.

Allow some time to pass, and when you feel ready, move your attention to a "neutral" person. Someone for whom you have no particular feelings one way or another. Perhaps someone at a local store or restaurant. Someone in an office across the hall. Someone to whom you've never paid any particular attention at all.

We often dismiss experiences that don't grab our initial attention. Once we categorize someone or some event as neutral, they are off the radar. So for these few minutes, picture this person, whose name you may not even know, knowing nothing about their lives or their difficulties, but recognizing that they are driven by the same human desires. Stay with the same wishes, the same phrases.

Next, move your attention to a difficult person. Don't start with the most difficult person in your life; that may be too much to ask. But find someone who challenges you, maybe someone you have a tense relationship with in your family, or a person in life who has annoyed you in some way. Now offer them the same phrases, the same intentions. Recognize that, in spite of any disagreements, whatever they've done was almost certainly driven by the same wishes for happiness, or ease, or peace of mind.

By wishing someone well, we're not condoning behavior, or putting a falsely positive spin on anything. We can still choose to push back, make changes, or even put someone out of our lives. When possible, though, we can do so with an understanding that while we may be completely at odds, we may see the world from an entirely different point of view, our goals as human begins are the same.

Thinking about a challenging person in this way can be overwhelming. If you find it too difficult, you might picture yourself at the same time. May we both be happy. May we both be safe. May we both live our lives with ease. You also can always return your intentions to only yourself, or to your breath. There's no need to force anything. Explore what is comfortable and uncomfortable, making whatever adjustments you need.

Traditionally, in ending, we offer these wishes to larger groups of people, recognizing that throughout the world, these are the same desires with which people live. You might turn your attention to all of the individuals that you've brought to mind; yourself, your benefactor and friend, a neutral person and a challenging one. May everyone in this group find peace, ease and well being. And then imagine the same for everyone outside the group you haven't yet thought of, recognizing the basic motivations behind the actions all people take, every day. Spend a few minutes with these more general thoughts, *may you all be happy, healthy, safe and at ease,* without trying to create any particular outcome in how you feel. If this ending feels too awkward, you might return to your family, picturing each member individually.

You can use these phrases throughout the day during moments when you find yourself stressed. Find a sense of peace with yourself without glossing over the rough spots and recognize flaws as they are. Ease your experience by searching for the line between working to improve yourself and belittling yourself for needing improvement in the first place. Life is challenging enough without self-judgment and abuse.

Skillful Communication with Children

We were walking up to the cash register and I felt myself get tense. I wanted to grab the two kids and march right through, but I had to pay first.

Last time was such a mess. Joey grabbed a toy from that annoying basket of crap they keep for impulse buys. So, without thinking, I snapped. "Put that back, we don't need it." So then his older brother Michael grabbed it from his hand, and I said, "Get your hands off of him." But then I realized he was only trying to get Joey to put the toy back. Joey started screaming and crying, and Michael started pushing him away from the toys and it was such an embarrassing mess.

This time, Joey immediately started reaching again. I took a few breaths. I turned to face the two of them, and quietly explained to Joey we weren't buying anything more today. And when Michael went to help him put it away, I thanked him but asked him to wait. Joey still started to get upset, but I was able to comfort him instead of riling up both of them.

It's been like that a lot. The calmer I stay, the calmer my kids stay. It seems obvious now, but it wasn't before. It's not always easy, but it helps.

∞

What does skillful communication mean? We've all seen it. You might be able to imagine a person you respect. What traits do you see when they interact with the world? Friendly, strong, funny, calm, compassionate, well spoken, or whatever else, their style often reflects a balance of inner strength, wisdom, and empathy.

Communication with children is an intricate dance for parents. We're always the grown-up—not a friend, not an equal. We set the ground rules, we uphold limits. We have the broader perspective. But while we maintain our place as the responsible adult, we also convey unconditional warmth and affection, collaborate when we can, and demonstrate an understanding that we are not infallible.

As well, our children observe and learn from our interactions with our spouse, neighbors, and out in the world. When we yell, our children yell. When we're nasty, sarcastic, or dismissive, our children learn those tendencies. When we shut down, don't listen, and lock onto a particular outcome, our children shut down as well.

If we approach them braced for the nightly homework battle, our children know what's coming. *"Why haven't you started? What's your excuse this time?"* Or it might be implied, your disappointment shimmering below the surface of the conversation, carried by your tone of voice.

It might be communicated in the way you enter the room and take over the situation. If your boss threw open the door to the office with the same attitude and posture, how would you respond? If they just walked in and, in a situation where you truly needed help figuring something out, took over without including you?

Your children are an equal part of the equation. You may speak in the wisest, calmest manner possible but they still yell and scream or refuse your help. But you can't control that right now. What you can do is manage your own response. What would best get this problem handled? What's a skillful approach for dealing with this confrontation?

As with any aspect of life, habits develop. An "easy" child without ADHD may grow up with positive feedback and endless latitude to debate rules and explore options. A challenging child may face strictness, demands, and criticism. Or you may treat the world one way, and your family another, reining yourself in outside the house, letting loose when you're home. Or vice versa.

Your child may chronically lose stuff. As they get older, the list becomes less trivial—first it was parts of toys and now it's jackets, a cell phone, the house keys. You try reasoning. You try yelling. Nothing changes, and this time their entire backpack is missing. Gone, all their books and half-completed homework and an expensive pair of running shoes.

You storm into their room to confront them. *"How could this happen again? We've talked about it over and over. Can't you see how much this costs us? Doesn't it matter to you that you have to do all your homework again? That's it. You're grounded until you've caught up on all the work you lost. Maybe now you'll get it."*

What's been communicated beyond your words? How close to a solution have you gotten? You've judged the situation and solved it, and your child hasn't even spoken yet. Or maybe they protested or made excuses. But then they probably started on their heels, off balance.

What back story have you created that is guiding this discussion? How open are you to other pictures of their future, or about yourself? You cannot get inside their brain and control them like a puppet. You may be frustrated, at wit's end, or feel lost. Acknowledging all that, what skillful action can you take next? What do you do habitually that has been useful, or not so useful?

You allow yourself a different way of responding when you create space between your thoughts and emotions and your reaction to them. Monitor all the frustration and tension in your body, and whatever is going on in your mind. Noticing any pressure from judgment and expectation and moving it to the side, pausing, what decision could you make next that might facilitate a different outcome?

Wherever your mind runs off to, past or future, you can practice noticing the diversion and coming back to the experience at hand. Right now, you're trying to figure out how to manage the lost backpack. You may absolutely need a new and improved long-term plan as well. But how would you advise a friend to act, *tonight?*

✿

Clear communication with a child with ADHD starts with a recognition of their biology. ADHD itself affects communication. It might seem intuitive that when we speak, the person we're addressing listens. ADHD often gets in the way of that simple transaction.

Attention-shifting problems prevent you from being heard as a parent—literally. If you don't make sure you have the full attention of a child with ADHD before you make a request, they probably won't hear you. Distractibility may come across as disinterest, or an attempt to tune a parent out.

Impulsivity may lead to things being said by a child without thinking. With ADHD, listening quietly—taking turns in conversation while a parent speaks—becomes immensely challenging. It may seem like disrespectful interruptions or willful ignoring, but much of it is driven by ADHD.

As the grown-up in the room, you adjust your expectations. You pause and collect yourself. But even if you're calmly starting at your best, you will still blow up at times. Pushed by a tantrum or silence, you'll be harsher or louder than you meant to be. Perfection is unattainable, but the possibility of honest reflection and following up to clarify ourselves is always available, and represent perhaps the keystone of skillful communication.

Communication with Grown-Ups

The art of communicating with teachers and people in the community raises the bar for staying calm and compassionate. Parents naturally want to see the best in their children. Loving them without reservation they may focus on easy moments and deny what the rest of the world is saying. *My child is wonderful and smart and well-rounded, and we have a great time building Legos,* even though his teacher says he cannot sit through class, or is too physical with his classmates. It may feel protective to make excuses. *I'm sure he'll grow out of it, he's a boy. That teacher is too harsh. My husband was the same way when he was a kid and he's doing fine.*

Your experiences and observations may be completely true, but maybe theirs are as well. And if there is an overall pattern, hiding from it doesn't help anyone. Again, early intervention is vital to child development, and erring on the side of seeking advice may avoid issues down the road.

Getting bad feedback from a teacher is upsetting. When you hear it, pause. Notice any tendency to circle the wagons. The adrenaline flows and mentally you recoil. *How dare you say anything about my child?* Focus on your breath. How much of what is being said could be true? Notice your feelings of reactivity, the mind shutting down in a haze of emotion. Is there even one sentence in the midst of the conversation that offers something useful?

Ask for a moment to collect yourself. And then listen. Seek clarification. Reflect on the conversation, and if you are too enmeshed to be rational, run it by someone who will provide you sound, truthful advice. Find someone without the self-protective instinct you have for your child, someone supportive but willing to give honest, direct feedback.

CONVERSATION MEDITATION

Communication expands on the mindfulness techniques you have started practicing—stepping out of autopilot, becoming less reactive, and learning your own mental tendencies. With any conversation or interaction, our expectations of the outcome influence how we hold ourselves, our choice of words, and our tone of voice. Pausing and listening, not forcing an immediate solution, we allow other plausible outcomes to emerge.

The path of any conversation is steered by much more than our words alone. Before we open our mouths to speak we often anticipate how the discussion will go, which affects what we choose to say and how we say it. Our nonverbal language, such as facial expression or posture, generally develops without our awareness and may tell more about our intention than the words we choose. We're offering an opportunity for explanation, but our skepticism is etched in our faces. Our ability to listen and respond is affected by our acute mental and physical states, as well as by years of experience through which we filter our lives. We'll hear things quite differently while we're relaxed and on vacation than when we're harried and walking in the door from work.

A communication style where you accept everything you hear and never state your needs is not the point. You're angry—that's real. There is a serious problem that needs solving—that's real as well. Communicating mindfully doesn't involve rolling over and giving up, it means keeping your own perspective yet empathetically noticing the viewpoint of another.

Somewhere in the middle is an opportunity to listen, to creatively problem solve, to engage your child in the discussion without escalating their fear. As always, underneath their anger, withdrawn sullen silence, or seeming apathy, below all of it they want what you want. They'd like to be happy and at ease, and that's what you picture for them as well.

A communication checklist:

- Pause and listen first
- Monitor your body language and tone
- Monitor your expectations and any predictions of what will come next
- When needed, take a few breaths—or take a break
- Pay full attention and create a situation where whomever you are talking to can do the same; stay away from other people, television, phones, computers, etc. while engaging in discussion.

Decisions, Decisions

So much has changed. I've stopped expecting that there's always something more to do. He's doing so much better in so many ways, it's easy to always think we have to work on something else, to push him more. It's easy to forget to be happy with everything we've accomplished already.

And I'm trusting him more. I'm letting him make more choices—and make mistakes, when I can. Sometimes I have to tell him what to do, of course. But a lot of the time I give him a chance. He messes up and we discuss what happened. Sometimes he gets in trouble and he doesn't argue the same way. He realizes there was a problem, and expects the consequence.

But even more often, he gets around to better choices. It may take him a while, but he gets there.

∽∾

From any single difficult behavior arises a string of choices: How do I manage it at home, at the grocery store, or at grandma's house? The answers are not always black and white, creating ambiguity which often escalates the tension, but some basic guidelines generally hold true. As a bottom line, all we can do each time we make a new decision is pause and make the best choice we see, with the tools and information we have at our disposal; when the moment has passed, reflect on what's happened; and then if needed, make adjustments, or make amends.

You're in the store and realize something needs to change. You're the one whose child is running around holding the gold-plated fishing pole. Now what? How do you start using mindfulness in your life? With the beginning exercises, pausing and paying attention. Without any direct effort, practicing these skills affects your moment to moment experience.

You start by settling yourself. Stressed, you're less likely to be at your best. You're also less likely to solve problems creatively. When simply aware, without entanglement, answers often become clear.

You seek the reality of the moment, cutting yourself some slack, and cutting your kids as much. Maybe there's something different to be done in your parenting, at school, or in medical treatment. Maybe there's something you can teach your children, some new concept or new approach that will help build their ability to self-regulate.

With awareness of your inner state, you don't react wildly, compelled by unconscious impulses. You become more aware of what is going on in your mind. When you're irritated, you know you're irritated, and when you're anxious, you know you're anxious. There's nothing forced about this, but there is an assumption that when you are more conscious of these inner experiences, you'll handle them with more skill.

You practice patience. When you grab for a solution without pausing, you often find the same one you've always tried, forcing a square peg in a round hole. Or maybe you try to motivate with honey, or with a big stick, when motivation isn't the underlying problem at all. Or blindly miss another option that might work better that has been staring you in the face all along.

At any time in life, you can notice your judgments, opinions, and constructions—the thumbnail sketches you've written about yourself, your family, or a situation. These thoughts might be true, and they might not. Noticing them, you let them go without getting stuck, and come back to your immediate reality.

You begin to observe, with clarity, conflicts with your child and her ADHD. Have you explored the difference between what you believe *should be* and what actually *is?* What are her true strengths and vulnerabilities? What are yours?

The long-term goal of helping build skills, manage ADHD, create relationships—all that stays the same. You're not giving up. But what are the basics facts, right now? Wanting your child to be motivated or less impulsive or more organized cannot alter anything this moment.

So you took a step. You let a behavior slide this time, or you took away TV time, or you resolved to call a family therapist for help. You made the best choice you could have right then, with the resources you had at your disposal and the information you understood. What happened next?

Mindfulness is not about doing anything *better* or *worse* than before. You can't do anything better *yesterday*. The following day you may realize it wasn't such a great way to act, or that the end result was not what you had hoped. You may believe it turned out to be just about the least skillful way you could have responded.

Some plan hasn't been working so far. You still argue all the time about school. Or maybe you get along great at home, but he still battles with other children. Remain open to the possibility that this time the outcome could be different. Maybe with patience the exact same routine leads somewhere completely different this time around, the lesson learned. And then again, maybe a wiser option would be choosing a new path entirely. Observe the outcomes of your behaviors and actions with all the compassion and objectivity you can muster, and then resolve to move forward again.

❧

Meditation is a technique to help see clearly. Our vision is distorted by all the random thoughts, reactions, emotions, fantasies, memories, and day-to-day chaos of our ordinary lives. Would you want to invest in an expensive stock based on such skewed information? Instead, we try to see past our filters and fog.

Having intention to do something without any expectation of a particular outcome is a somewhat quirky concept. I'm going to sit in meditation, do my best to stay focused, expect distractions endlessly, and I may or may not find myself relaxed this time around. You can try it out with commonplace activities, too. For example, you might be working toward your child making his bed every morning. You create a plan, observe, and take a breath when the bed is, yet again, a complete mess. And then come back to the goal, make an adjustment, and try again.

Train a sense that you'll continue to persevere to find solutions and, at the same time, let go of any expectations that everything will fall instantly into place. There's no guarantee that *this* plan will change everything right now. Each step of the way, aiming to be aware and accepting of the ups and downs of life, without expecting anything different.

Mindfulness Tools in Everyday Life

I'm a screamer, and I come from generations of screamers. But I'm working on it. Now I pause and try to remember to take a breath. Most of the time, I catch myself. And my household is so much quieter. My kids are less argumentative. Instead of shouting ourselves in circles, we talk. Even when they get in trouble, they don't argue so much.

⟡

While you'll still encounter moments of joy, sorrow, stress, and relaxation throughout your life, practicing mindfulness allows a fresh perspective. Through steady attention and self-care, you'll cultivate a new way of living for yourself and your family. The most specific goal of mindfulness has been said to be the elimination of suffering, or, rather, the promotion of happiness and well-being—which will mean something different to every family.

Practicing mindfulness and an increased sense of well-being go together for people. How come? Various psychological characteristics have been teased out of the mix by researchers, specific traits that correlate with the benefits people report. These traits help explain the nuances of what people develop as they practice mindfulness consistently. They also represent qualities that enhance parenting, especially when dealing with a child with ADHD, and have reciprocal benefits for the entire family. Here's a summary of some skills that can develop if you continue with the exercises:[5]

- Paying attention to moment-to-moment experiences.
- Getting out of autopilot.
- Noticing and labeling internal states as they happen.
- Responding instead of reacting to experience.
- Moving beyond reactive judgment and bias.
- Acting with intention.

❧

Not everything is going to change in a day, after reading one chapter explaining mindfulness. You still may find yourself herding children toward the door, but thinking about what you need to do after the kids leave for school. Or maybe doing your chores, but planning what you'll say to your spouse at dinner. Or while you're eating dinner with your family, you may be thinking about a problem at work... all of which, on a basic level, means you likely miss out on a lot of fun stuff in life and with your kids. But through your growing mindfulness practice, maybe you'll notice yourself off planning or ruminating earlier than before and once or twice even catch yourself and return.

Pausing, you also can choose to respond, rather than react out of uncontrolled frustration. Lost in distraction, living on autopilot, means you are not paying full attention to the infinite choices you're making every day. You now have the opportunity to cultivate the ability to address day-to-day challenges calmly and proactively, instead of falling back on habitual reactions. When you practice meditation, you develop the capacity to notice an emotional reaction—I'm feeling angry—and not act on it immediately. You have started to create a space to find your own clarity, and while you may still decide to do the exact same thing you've always done, perhaps you will choose otherwise.

You can select where to place your attention. You might start with your child, focusing only on him a few minutes each day, pulling your mind out of distraction. Behavioral change often follows when parents pay dedicated attention for a little time each day.

Through mindfulness, you have the opportunity to cultivate less habitual judging of things, the endlessly categorizing of experiences into good, bad, better, or worse. This ability, as we reviewed, contrasts with discernment. You set goals and try to change things, but without as much internal angst. It doesn't matter what you *should* have done *before;* all you can control is what you do *next*.

You continue to seek the reality or the "bare facts" of a situation, without adding biases or reactive judgments. Problems that seemed concrete often turn out to be fluid. Thoughts like *my child will never, ever be different than this,* or *there is nothing I can do to change this behavior* feel like unblinking reality. However, neither statement is necessarily true. What feels solid and fixed often originates from unconscious rumination and mental habit. With an ability to be more responsive, and without falling back on old habits, you instead pause and make conscious, skillful choices. New possibilities begin to exist.

When fear rules your thoughts, it controls your attention. It grabs hold and won't let go. All you see are the unsettling fantasies, nothing more. You say and do things to modulate the emotions, to try and make it better—even when the event itself is long gone, or yet to come.

Treating your kids and yourself with compassion in the deepest sense is a recognition that not every slipup and misbehavior stems from actual intent. Difficult behaviors related to ADHD—from overt impulsivity, to trouble with teachers, to more subtle challenges with disorganization, motivation, time management, and misplacing belongings—are almost certainly not intentional. Once again, your children are trying to find some peace and well-being, and ADHD is thwarting their efforts.

Left unattended, the daily chaos of life perpetuates itself. Short of a crisis, when do you decide to stop, make a proactive decision, and try something new? How you live, how you behave, how much TV you watch, how you eat—as hard as these patterns are to change it's your choice to continue the status quo or not.

You may choose to pick up the tools of mindfulness at any time. But don't blame yourself for what you've felt or done before, or what you feel now. You've been happy or sad because you've been happy or sad.

You've made the best choices you could, with the knowledge you had. That's all any of us does, every day.

Most children need some extra help or behavioral modification at some point in their lives. It doesn't mean you screwed up. *I should have handled that better, my child shouldn't act that way, that person over there thinks I'm the worst parent ever.* Noticing any of that type of thinking, you practice letting it go—that's the voice of judgment again, not reality.

However as much you are struggling, however much you feel like you messed up, your motivation was true. Whatever step—or misstep—you took you were trying your best. Let go of any effort to force your life into a perfect picture. Maybe you're stressed. Maybe your child has ADHD. Those are simple facts. Try to address each with all the compassion you can muster. And then use the mindfulness tools to find ease in life and in your family.

Standing in place, we subtly but endlessly shift our weight to remain upright. There is a constant need for corrections to maintain balance. And so it is in life—exploring when to lean forward or duck back, and myriad other moment-to-moment adjustments. Cultivating a dynamic platform of strength and stability, you make clear-sighted, proactive choices that build your own resilience, your child's ability to self-regulate, and a foundation for a family full of health and well-being.

◈

Explore the exercises offered throughout this chapter at your own pace. Return to them whenever you'd like, perhaps trying one out for several days or weeks. Set aside a specific time each day, such as when your kids are getting on the bus, or you have a lunch break, or right after bedtime. Create an electronic reminder for yourself, or make a note on your calendar.

The following six-week program exploring mindfulness reflects the way the mindfulness-based stress reduction program is typically taught. Each week, exercises from the book are referenced for your review. Do your best to follow the suggested outline, and when you lose track or forget, come back to it again. It is adapted from the original program offered at the University of Massachusetts, as well as a parent-specific version created by Amy Saltzman, M.D. (who mentored me in starting my own classes). This outline is meant as an overview. Teachers also offer in-person programs throughout the country, and the world; a partial list is available at the Center for Mindfulness, University of Massachusetts website.

Week 1:

- Spend dedicated time with your children once each day, focused only on an activity as it happens (page 57).
- Sitting or lying down, guide yourself through a body scan meditation (page 82) once daily. Commit to a time, scheduling it when you are alert and less likely to fall asleep.
- Pay attention to the "voice of judgment" as you encounter it throughout the week, internal commentaries about your own thoughts or behavior, or comparing something in the world to how it "should" be, or any other place you stumble over it (page 94).
- Once during the week—or once a day—eat a snack or meal with similar attention, focusing on eating, pausing, and deciding when to move to the next bite instead of mindlessly consuming your food (page 91).

Week 2:

- Continue to spend time with your children each day in which they lead the activity and you follow. As well, find one pleasurable experience each day and bring your full attention to it, choosing anything from your first sip of coffee in the morning to a date night with your spouse.
- Focus on your breath during daily meditation (page 67). Without trying to force yourself to relax, or expecting yourself to block out all thoughts, practice sitting and letting your mind quiet down. Release any sense of effort or judgment for these few minutes, as best you can.
- Pay attention to your schedule, and how you use your time each day this week. What could be juggled to carve out a few minutes for yourself? Where are you overscheduled in ways that you can change? How would you like to be spending your time? If you cannot change your schedule, could you find even a moment to pause and step out of the mental chaos? (page 83)

Week 3:

- While continuing to focus on simple, pleasurable experiences in life and with your children, start to pay attention to unpleasant or stressful experiences. Observe how you feel emotionally and physically. And perhaps notice when your thoughts run into the future, or remain caught in the past. Without forcing or repairing anything, staying focused on the unfolding of your experience as it happens, and your responses.

- Continue your daily meditation, focusing on the breath. As you sit, pay attention to body sensations, emotions, and thoughts as they arise. Notice your reaction to them, any urge to move away or fix them or reject them out of hand. And then, for these few minutes, return to simply observing (page 174).

- Schedule pauses several times during the day. Create them as reminders in your calendar, or post yourself notes in one or two places in the house. Or stop for a moment each day before leaving home, and before entering the front door again. Or choose whatever else fits for you (page 98).

Week 4:

- Practice pausing throughout each day. Instead of reacting instantly, out of habit, take a breath. Stop. Notice what's actually going on around you. And then, with intention, choose a next step (page 98).

- Pay attention to how you feel and act when stressed. How does your body feel? What effect does stress have on your mind, or on your emotional state, and how long does it all continue? (page 64)

- Focus on compassion, in life and in your meditation (page 103). Choose concepts that feel natural to you and even in a stressful moment, use them to bring yourself back. *My child is making a scene, I'm getting embarrassed and frustrated. In spite of the mess, and regardless of how it looks from the outside, we're both trying our best to be settled and at ease.* Start with yourself, and then move outward with thoughts for people in the world around you.

Week 5:

- Continue to practice pausing. When you feel yourself revved up or mentally out of control in the midst of a crazy day, step aside. Even for just a minute—for ten or fifteen breaths—let your mind settle again.
- Focus on communication with your children (page 109). Notice any expectations (*I'm going to say this, and then he's going to say...*) or compulsions to create a particular outcome. While maintaining a clear sense of your role as a parent, also notice how you carry yourself, and your own habits and perceptions. Pay attention to what you model for them in conversation, and in conflict resolution. Strive each time to listen, pause, and only then respond.
- Continue to focus on compassion in your daily meditation. You deserve to feel happy, strong, and at ease. Everyone else does, too. Even while protecting yourself, or emphatically disagreeing with someone, recognizing that behind even an ill-conceived action typically is a desire for well-being (page 103).

Week 6:

- In ending your formal six week schedule, choose whatever meditation fits for you to practice. Sitting, walking, or standing (page 154). Breathing or focusing on compassion. Practicing yoga. Whatever you select, commit to your chosen activity once daily. Or maybe take ten minutes a few times a day to meditate, to manage your stress, settle your mind, and cultivate self-awareness and compassion.
- Protect time to take care of yourself. Go for a run—but focus only on the run. Play tennis, read a book, or go to a movie. Do the dishes and focus on the dishes, not on the to-do list. Cultivate equanimity and well-being in yourself, and you bring those benefits to the family.
- Pay attention to smooth and pleasant family time. Protect it, schedule it, and, if needed, create it, fifteen minutes or half an hour during which your child chooses the activity, and you follow.
- Continue to practice pausing and responding, instead of reacting out of habit, when stressed or facing challenges.

- Commit to a plan for the future that includes daily meditation and a general focus on mindfulness. Place a reminder on your calendar several months out to see if you've kept up. Find a couple of words, maybe two or three, that represent the traits you'd like to develop. Calmness. Wisdom. Humor. Strength. Compassion. Joy. Write them down somewhere, and when tumult takes over in life, return to them.

The Foundations of ADHD Care

So now we move forward to intervention for ADHD. What can you offer a child with ADHD that manages the symptoms and builds a sense of well-being? How do you develop your own strength and resilience? And what can you do for your family?

Support for children with ADHD falls into three broad areas of life—home, school, and medical approaches. In any of these areas, decisions become clearer with an understanding of ADHD, from its underlying biology to the effects of executive function and impulse control problems on children.

First we'll talk about life at home. Research shows that children with ADHD are more likely to thrive when receiving positive rather than negative feedback—but it can be difficult to balance positive discipline with the needs of a child with ADHD. They require clear limit setting and an emphasis on routines. They require that adults scale down their expectations and develop long-term goals balanced by a clear view of a child's actual abilities.

When it comes to school, we cannot expect kids with ADHD to manage their schoolwork, sit in a chaotic classroom, or learn new information at the same pace and with the same supports as peers. Instead, we need to create alternative methods to help children excel.

Last are medical interventions. ADHD is a biological condition, and medications address an inherent physical difference in the brain. ADHD medication improves self-regulation, and, in spite of how they are often portrayed, side effects tend to be less significant than the risks inherent in untreated ADHD. Various alternative interventions have some evidence behind them as well, but not as replacements for ADHD medication.

Reviewing all these different possibilities, some of which you may have encountered, many of which you may have strong beliefs about, may be stressful for you. Changing a belief or a personal habit is hard. Trying new things at home can be disruptive and difficult. School may be a constant battle, and you may feel that the system is not on your side. Medications may feel uniquely terrifying.

Using the mindfulness tools, pause as you feel your stress level rise. Notice any escalating thoughts and emotions. Notice when your mind leaps into the future with fantasies of what might happen next. Notice reflexive reactions or beliefs. *Routines will never work, we already tried rewards, his teacher doesn't listen to me, medications will change him forever.* Instead of getting snagged, focus back on your breathing, for a minute, or for five or fifteen. Step by step, come back to this moment only, choosing what seems like the best *next* step, nothing more.

PART III

Promoting Well-Being: Comprehensive Support for Families and Children

CHAPTER 7

Behavior: Avoiding the "No, David" Approach

*W*hat actually improves behavior for kids with ADHD? My clinical experience confirms what the research reveals, that emotionally supportive but consistently firm parenting works best for families with ADHD. What I've seen throughout my career is that these simple but quite challenging to implement concepts lead to a ripple effect. The longer parents stand by them, the easier life becomes. No matter what may feel intuitive or may have become habit in any particular home, ADHD requires a return to these evidence-based basics.

As mundane as these parenting fundamentals may sound on the surface, they are hard to maintain. Praise that may have been effective for a sibling may not be enough to encourage appropriate behavior in your child with ADHD. Because of this, parents may give up on using targeted positive feedback to affect change at home. Also, ADHD-related behaviors require near-constant correction for some kids, creating a background hum of "don't touch that, don't run into the street, get back over here and finish your dinner." A tough-to-break cycle of negativity often follows.

Many parents were raised in strict environments themselves, held to high standards that, when broken, led directly to punishment. But raising a child with ADHD may require letting go of this picture of parenting, as it may provoke more problems than it solves. Instead, a balance can be found where a parent can firmly uphold limits while creating an overall home environment that seeks out and emphasizes a child's successes.

Studies show that therapeutic interventions aimed at parents affect ADHD symptoms more than when therapists interact only with children. We work toward an environment where both parents coordinate *to implement these proven behavioral techniques. Individual behavioral therapy for children is most effective for related issues, such as helping with poor self-esteem or anxiety, building organizational skills, and promoting healthy family relationships.*

Hearing that parenting affects ADHD may sound as if you've done something wrong or should be doing a better job. It's not that. You've always done the best you can and there's always something new to learn and try. The balance is being open to change without lamenting the fact that you haven't been perfect before.

⌦

Start at the Start

If you handed me a basketball and offered me one million dollars to hit ten consecutive free throws today, there is almost no chance I'd succeed. If you gave me six months or a year to practice, I might. Motivation alone doesn't change our capacity to achieve, so behavior management starts with an objective look at your child's skills.

Outside of horror movies, children are not inherently bad, and their issues do not stem from lack of effort. They may misbehave, talk back, not listen, skip homework, or hit other children. But behind their behavior is the same simple goal that drives all of us—a desire to be happy.

So, a child sees a toy they want. They make a mistaken assumption, perhaps true in the short-term, that having that toy will make them happy. Then they knock down another child and grab the toy. Why? On a basic level, the reason is simple. They want the toy and don't have another means to get it. And they doesn't know how to handle the frustration of not having it.

The underlying issue is a child who does not have the capacity to do anything else. In spite of knowing the rules, kids with poor frontal lobe function are impulsive and act before thinking. They may know immediately they've blown it and made a mistake, but the act itself occurred before thought.

Change Begins with You

I'm much happier when I remind myself that his behavior isn't always personal, it's biological. It's who he is. He's still responsible for himself, of course. But some of his behavior is his ADHD. I know he's smart enough to get A's, but intellect isn't everything you need for good grades. He's getting A's and B's this year, and he's starting to take more responsibility for his work.

⟳∞⟲

While biology drives ADHD, parenting choices have a profound impact in modulating the symptoms. You didn't cause the ADHD, but you do influence the outcome. This fact probably feels both liberating and overwhelming.

Parenting basics may seem like common-sense guidelines, and they are. But where other children may respond well to a wider range of parenting styles, children with ADHD require parents to more consistently adhere to these basics. Until children have the capacity to monitor their own behavior, create their own routines, and manage their own responsibilities, they will need these supports. And a child with ADHD is going to require them for several years more than their peers.

As a parent of a child with ADHD, you're being held to a high standard. You have to stay positive in the face of slow progress when a child does not consistently do what you think best. You might stick to reward systems over months or years even while behavior improves only incrementally. And then problem behaviors return the moment you take a break—didn't he learn anything? You restructure your household around ADHD, live differently than you pictured, and still the demands escalate.

So you rally and create a new routine and set up a new behavioral reward system and vow to be consistent in limit setting. After a while, life intervenes and you drift back toward whatever feels easiest for you, and things go downhill again. It's not right or wrong, it's what happens. Styles of parenting grow out of ADHD triage.

A child's inability to follow routines, impulsiveness, poor listening, irritability, or poor communication challenges parents, regardless of their intentions. Research shows that parents of children with ADHD tend toward punitive parenting. It makes sense, as they have children who require redirection in order to be safe, do their work, get ready for bed, and complete countless other details of the day. Their children do not respond as easily to praise alone when learning new behaviors; they have ADHD, so they struggle. Yet parenting that leans too far in the punitive direction only exacerbates ADHD in the long haul.[1]

Parents of kids with ADHD struggle to maintain routines and consistency in setting limits. You put in the effort to establish routines, and then your kids don't follow them. Or it takes them a long time to adjust...and when you stop monitoring, your children forget again. Influenced by all of this, parents of kids with ADHD report less of a sense of control over their lives, which leads to less creative problem solving.[2]

COULD YOU HAVE ADHD?

Parents of children with ADHD are several times more likely than other parents to have ADHD themselves. Adults with ADHD struggle with routines, time management, organization and planning, and sometimes even impulsivity and emotional reactivity.

As you'd approach your child with compassion while addressing their needs, look at yourself the same way. Notice your own habits. It could be upsetting to hear or validating to discover that you have ADHD symptoms, but you either have ADHD symptoms, or you don't. Let go of any judgment that arises.

A free screening tool created through the World Health Organization is available on line, or you can contact your doctor with questions. If you think you may have ADHD, follow through to get evaluated. You will support not only yourself, but your family and your children by seeking a solution.

⚮

Parenting style matters in ADHD. While this is not the same as saying parenting causes ADHD, different methods of parenting tend to be more effective and more likely to minimize symptoms. Behavioral progress happens when parents take the lead, stick by new systems, and remain patient with their children. Children learn new skills and take control of their lives at some point, but through most of childhood, parents create the broader framework for change.

But parenting a child who cannot follow rules well or maintain routines, or who impulsively reacts and get angry all day long, takes its toll. The strain of managing behavior leads to elevated anxiety levels, an increased risk of depression, and impacts marriages. The angst of making difficult decisions about school, help at home, or medical interventions, gnaws. Well-meaning, loving parents pour themselves into caring for their children and become exhausted.

Taking care of children begins with carving out and protecting your own internal resources. Your children do come first. But if you are burned out or overwhelmed, it limits what you can give to them. If your marriage is strained and your relationship with your spouse chronically tense, it affects your children. When you are too harried to notice creative solutions, old habits remain entrenched.

If you expect yourself to be a perfect parent, you'll fail. The reality is, you will make some choices seeking happiness and peace of mind for yourself that work, and some that don't. Your child's attempts at seeking happiness and peace of mind will sometimes work and sometimes won't. And your view and your child's may often be at odds, as what you decide is best may not exactly match your child's preference. He wants to go to a pool party instead of working on a research paper and doesn't care a whole lot about his physics project today.

The mindfulness techniques you have been reading about refer to activities that support you, as a parent. They focus on a bigger picture, affecting how you manage the daily challenges life presents. You cannot do everything "right" as a parent, or depend on a uniform, cookie-cutter approach to "fixing" life, since there is no one perfect solution. Instead, you can cultivate balance and wisdom, which allow you to manage family life to the best of your ability.

Mindfulness builds the skills you need, clearing the way for an objective look at ADHD and at your individual child's strengths and weaknesses. Chronic stress changes the quality of your interactions and limits your ability to accept life's ups and downs. Managing stress starts with just a few minutes a day, a pause to settle the mind and step back out of the chaos of a busy life. When you feel better, become a little less reactive, or find novel solutions to problems, your children's behavior and happiness often follow. As the fog lifts, you may find a smoother path to the future.

> ### REACHING OUT
>
> Skillful parenting often arises from recognizing when you need sup-
> port. If you're ever feeling like you are going under, reaching out for
> help is a sign of strength. Working with a therapist to address your
> own concerns or improve your marriage can make a huge difference
> for your children.

Basic Parenting Guidelines

Parenting is an art informed by research and science. We can
describe in broad strokes what works for children with ADHD, but
the details will always vary. There are few hard-and-fast rules, and
rarely one right answer to managing behavior.

Studies of parenting and ADHD point at several skills that improve
parent-child relationships and children's behavior. An emphasis on
positive feedback compensates for children's ADHD-driven experiences of the world, the constant corrections children face. Structure
and routine can help with executive function deficits. And paying
attention to what you model as an adult is another general foundation
of parenting.

What is presented here is meant as an overall framework, not
an instruction manual for every issue that may arise. The basics of
parenting a child with ADHD integrate the research with the reali-
ties of home life. You want day-to-day logistics to run smoothly.
You want your child to be happy, to have friends, and to succeed
academically. By remaining open and balancing the basic guidelines with what works for your family, you'll make adjustments and
address problems creatively while meeting the individual needs of
your child.

1. Praise and Reward

Families of children with ADHD often fall into the "No, David" trap.
No, David!, by David Shannon, is an illustrated children's book with
few words. In the pictures, a rambunctious child runs and jumps and
impulsively gets into trouble. David's mother repeats "No, David"
throughout the book—appropriately, one might guess, as David needs

to be kept safe. But "No, David" is an attitude that can become a lifestyle.

Kids suffer in the long run if they hear all the "no's" from adults without enough notice of their successes. Children with ADHD need guidance and limit-setting from adults as much, if not more, than other children. Yet children with ADHD get redirection about their off-task or inappropriate behavior all day long, far more than smiles and "yes's" and encouragement. It's not a surprise when self-esteem and self-confidence erode over time.

Children require positive feedback from the world, a sense that, whatever mistakes they make, they are successful at something and valued by others. Praise can modify behavior; you can cultivate the opposite of the behavior you are trying to eliminate. Though it won't fix everything, it is another starting point (along with spending planned time with your children) for many intensive behavioral plans.

As you set out to recognize and comment on small successes, you may find that, lost in your own distractions, you miss out on these passing moments. You stew in your mind, still angry your child missed the bus again, and the morning washes past. But even in the midst of the most challenging situations, there usually are times when your child succeeds and behaves appropriately.

Start by emphasizing success in daily life and praising the opposite of the behaviors you would like to avoid. Children are motivated by their parents' approval. Targeted praise often modifies behavior all on its own, as well as balancing the corrections children with ADHD have likely been receiving.

Sometimes, behavior changes through this shift in emphasis. Handing your child a dish to help set the table, you thank them for the great work before they have a chance to get it wrong. You compliment the first moments that two siblings are playing together, before they begin to bicker. Even when behaviors don't immediately improve through targeted praise, the balance shifts back toward healthy ego development and easier relationships.

Another way of maintaining a positive, nurturing perspective is through rewards such as sticker charts for younger children, and more complicated reward systems for older ones. Often called "token economies," these systems allow kids to earn points toward a longer-term goal, and in some cases permit losing points as well.

BUILDING A REWARD SYSTEM

- **Choose a target behavior.** Initially, pick only one or two behaviors you would like to change. When possible, set positive goals; for example, "talk nicely to grownups" can be used instead of "do not talk back." Set children up for success by narrowing your focus to something within their reach. For systems to succeed, children must earn points far more than they miss them, so start small. As behaviors improve, you can gradually modify the program.

- **Choose something that will motivate your child—and that you can repeat again, in some format, down the road.** Common, inexpensive rewards may be stickers in younger children, or for older children treats like choosing a movie, media time, or small toys or games. If you set the bar too high from the start—like earning a new computer—what will you use next time around?

When stickers no longer motivate younger children, larger rewards should be earned over several days or, in older children, weeks. A certain number of "points"—perhaps a week's worth at first—qualify for the reward. Success should be based on a total number of points, not a consecutive number of days, allowing a child to continue earning toward their reward even when they "mess up" early in the week.

You also may consider breaking the day into smaller parts when children are struggling to earn their points; children might earn stickers or points for before and after lunch separately, for example.

- **Establish the rules for your children.** During a quiet time, sit down with your child and explain the new system, emphasizing their strengths, and that the system itself is not a punishment. Make sure that all the adults and children involved in the plan understand the expectations.

- **Prominently display your child's progress.** As an alternative to a paper chart displaying stickers or check marks, you can use a token jar to keep track, filling it with something like pennies or marbles. Comment on their success and praise progress frequently.

- **Reevaluate often.** If a reward system falls apart, pause and reassess. Are the expectations clear and consistently upheld? Is the time span small enough? Does your child want the selected prize? Parents often give up on reward systems when they really only need adjustments. Reward systems also sometimes take not weeks but months to affect change, especially with ADHD, and require a lot of modification, persistence, and patience.

You already know children with ADHD have difficulty with both remembering routines and with motivation. Reward systems, displayed prominently and often in multiple locations in the house, can nudge them in the appropriate direction. This is different from bribery, which is coercing someone to misbehave. You want to build self-esteem and shift the balance of your relationship away from the "No, David" style of correction and negativity.

2. The Power of Routine

Routine refers both to how you typically do things as a parent, and to the structure you create for your children. Monitor the routines you create at home, such as how you make requests or how you follow up, keeping in mind that executive function and attention problems directly affect parenting. For example, between distractibility and the hyper-focus often experienced by kids with ADHD, kids struggle to place their attention where it's needed. You walk past their room and call, "Dinner in five minutes!" and fifteen minutes go by—and the Lego castle is closer to completion but your child hasn't moved closer to the table.

A child with fluid attention abilities can rapidly move back and forth—someone's speaking, dinner soon, got it, and back to the Legos. For the average child with ADHD the request never fully registers. Maybe he notices someone speaking in the background, but the actual words were not heard, so he never responds. It may appear intentionally oppositional. Therefore, basic first step to getting things done is making sure that you have a child's full attention before making a request. Enter the room, find a natural break in their play, draw their focus to you, and then speak to them.

Difficulties with working memory prevent children from following mental lists. A casual request to take the garbage out, turn off the hose, and close the garage door falls apart halfway out the door. Between distractibility and poor working memory, the list is gone. He may be equally frustrated and at a loss—and make excuses or disappear. But he didn't choose to forget, he didn't have the skills to remember. So, you learn to keep requests simple, one thing at a time, until he proves that he can handle more complicated tasks.

Children with ADHD require household routines that consider executive function problems. Some skills can be taught: A step-by-step approach to tidying a bedroom breaks this surprisingly complex assignment into more manageable parts.

At other times you teach coping mechanisms, adaptations kids learn to compensate for their ADHD. Consistent morning, bedtime, and homework plans teach a life skill and help the household move smoothly. Without them most children with ADHD won't keep track of these responsibilities mentally, and parents end up micromanaging—did you brush your teeth, use the toilet, wash your hands, put the towel back on the rack...

Instead, you can create lists for common routines, and then steer your child back to checking them—literally post them around the house, using pictures for children who cannot read. In place of asking each detail, you remind them, 'Is the list done?' until finally they've learned the habit of maintaining and following a to-do list. This simple habit will go a long way at home, school, and in the workplace one day.

BED TIME: GETTING FROM A TO Zzzzz

Between compliance issues and the relative high incidence of sleep disturbances in kids with ADHD, good "sleep hygiene" becomes even more important than for other children. Even when there is a true sleep disturbance, the first steps toward management typically begin with establishing a consistent sleep routine (although other plans may be needed in the long run).

Children benefit from having the same bedtime, night after night, with calming activities proceeding lights out, like reading books or taking a bath—not playing video games or jumping on a trampoline.

Sleep habits, such as children expecting a parent to lie in their bed with them, or getting up to join parents in bed, easily perpetuate themselves. The easiest way to avoid these issues is to discourage them from the start. This is often easier said than done, and more detailed advice for this intricate and challenging area of parenting can be found in resources such as Dr. Marc Weissbluth's book *Healthy Sleep Habits, Happy Child*.

You can use the reward systems mentioned earlier to support almost any routine. They focus behavior change on success, motivate children to engage with a new system when they otherwise might resist, and create an incentive for children who are likely less motivated than their parents to put in the effort to break their old habits.

3. Limits Are a Teaching Tool

The next step is establishing a clear balance between all your praise and reward with emphatic, clear limit-setting. Neither functions well without the other. Children require a secure, supportive relationship with their parents, and praise directs behavior—to a point. Kids require consistent teaching of skills, redirection, and discipline, but again, not to exclusion of warmth and affection.

Children with ADHD struggle to self-regulate. Upholding limits and routines not only helps your household run smoothly but builds the executive function and related abilities that are required for your child to thrive as an adult. Maintaining clear boundaries that cause your children some consternation is *not* poor parenting. Life skills such as emotional resiliency and self-restraint build from an environment with consistent, clear limits.

While maintaining this perspective, help your child understand ADHD—that it has nothing to do with intelligence, or being bad, or defining who he is. Emphasizing his successes, frame ADHD-related challenges as just ADHD: *So many people with ADHD have the problem you're having with remembering your books. What plan can we create to make it easier for you?* Instead of, *You've got to stop forgetting your books, we've been talking about this for years.*

Without overfilling your child's schedule, cultivate activities in which he thrives. Find some aspect of life that comes naturally like art, sports, dance or whatever else, and let it happen. At the same time, do not make every moment of the schedule part of an intricate master plan. Continue to value unstructured time and play.

4. Monitor Your Own Consistency

Like the stress cycle, some patterns at home self-perpetuate. Children require more structure, more positive feedback to maintain motivation, and lots of flexible problem solving, and then ADHD pushes parents away from these tendencies. ADHD causes caregivers to correct their children a lot, and a child's variable response to discipline may in turn promote less consistency in their parents. But we also see that punitive or inconsistent parenting exacerbates behavioral issues in ADHD, which further wears down parents.

If you're not paying attention, these prolonged habits can become entrenched. Methods for managing behavior evolve all on their own, influenced by your upbringing but filtered through your experience. To build flexibility in your responses, continue the practice of "listen, breathe, respond," pausing and reflecting before proceeding.

Empty requests—ones made without backing yourself up—tell children that they can avoid things they don't want to do. If you ask something, do you follow through? It's often best to say nothing at all rather than ask for something you cannot properly enforce, so do not ask questions that are really statements. When you say, *"Will you help clear the table?"* do you actually mean *"Please clear the table now?"*

Consistency between caregivers also is vital. When two spouses have different standards, some children become confused, and others learn early on to play their parents against each other. While one parent pushes a child to follow rules, the other stands back and lets more infractions slide, creating a mixed message and sowing discord. With two different styles for managing behavior at home, ADHD symptoms may worsen and behavior will be slower to change. Involving teachers, babysitters, nannies, grandparents, or whomever else supervises your children in setting consistent expectations supports healthy development as well.

5. Ignore What You Can Ignore

Beyond the inviolate rules of life you define for your household, there often needs to be a behavioral triage that prioritizes what issues must be addressed versus those that can wait. Right now, today, what is the most pressing problem? Hitting other children—that has to stop first. No throwing tantrums around homework—maybe that's what has to be resolved instead. The rest might have to slide in the short run. A sloppy room, misplaced socks—these lesser issues may best move to the bottom of the list. Your child is not going to jump up and start cleaning her room right away and this may not be a crisis; it's a messy room, and not a danger to anyone.

Children with ADHD, however, don't get a free pass to misbehave. While ADHD explains many problem behaviors, this explanation shouldn't become a crutch. You still maintain standards of behavior, tempered, perhaps, by the reality of their symptoms.

Likewise, adults should not use ADHD as an excuse to disregard misbehavior. Even with ADHD, children eventually can be expected to treat others well, not be aggressive, speak appropriately to adults. It all comes down to balance. Recognizing what is driven by ADHD, you still set down clear rules about behaviors that are not ever appropriate.

Starting with the most disruptive behaviors, such as hitting, work on a behavioral plan. What might you accept as tolerable, while you address bigger concerns? What behavioral problems might you put aside for a stretch?

Your child rises from their chair for the eleventh time during dinner after you have asked her to remain seated every night for the last several years. Your blood pressure rises and your jaw aches, and you want to lash out. And at the same time...what are they experiencing? Can they, at this point in their life, really sit still? Can you more accurately match your expectations to their skills?

Choose what you'd like to change first for your child, and ignore the rest as much as possible. Not using ADHD as an excuse, continue to teach responsibility but let go of whatever you can at the same time. When a behavior is not dangerous, pause before responding. Think, is there something to be gained from a reaction this time around? Could you take a breath, and let it pass? Right now, you might be working on not talking back to adults, so hanging her coat on the hook may have to wait.

Notice your reaction, the frustration and anger, the sense that this moment isn't what it "should" be like, and then focus on the situation at hand. Uncover any tendency to push for more improvement, all the time. Maybe he's a B student right now, when last year he got C's. Maybe he remains over-talkative and impatient—but no longer fights with other children as much.

6. Consequences Should Be Immediate

As we've discussed, praise is rarely enough to change behavior all on its own. Parents need recourse, a way to uphold the rules. Most create a system that emphasizes time outs or removal of privileges. If you'd like,

offer one chance to change behavior—"I'm going to count to three"—
and that's it. Practice reserve. Without raising your voice, start a time
out, or stick to the consequences you have defined.

Children in general learn from immediate consequences, since
their brains aren't set up to connect the dots between past, present, and
future. Children with ADHD are delayed even more in this type of
thinking. A nine year old with ADHD may plan and consider for the
future like a five or six year old.

Your child pushes someone on the playground. "That's it, no
television tonight" is too abstract a response for most young children,
as later that night they'll be angry they've lost their privileges and
have no strong connection with why, even if you explain it again.
For a younger child the sequence probably feels more like, *Oops, I
hit someone, hmm, Mom's angry but nothing much happened.* And then
later that night, *This stinks, why can't I watch TV? I didn't do anything
wrong.*

Even as they get older, kids with ADHD do not learn much from
a punishment far removed from the event. Sent to their room, in a few
moments distractibility kicks in and they are happily playing. If they
lose a privilege at bedtime for a behavior that happened at lunch, there
isn't a concrete connection. To a child, it does not feel like discipline
anymore, it's a random frustrating event.

In addition to time outs, consequences can include loss of privileges,
the removal of a particular toy, or no media time. As well, ignoring
misbehavior can be a particularly useful response to a problem behavior,
because for many children getting no attention at all is even worse than
the negative attention received during punishment. Behaviors persist if
they are useful in some way—such as getting a grown-up's attention—
and decrease when they are not as useful. If a preschooler bites, after a
brief reprimand for whomever did the biting, you can lavish attention
on the other child alone.

7. Consequences—the Calm Way

While trying to discipline or control a distressing situation, you are also
training children in conflict resolution. They learn from your behavior
even while you're trying to affect theirs. Yelling and screaming teach
that the loudest voice wins. It's a short-term solution—you gain control.
But while it might work when preventing a child from running into the

street, it is a long-term loss when your child mimics the same tools with family and peers.

For example, time outs don't always work so smoothly at the start, and children may need direct supervision to stay in place. If your child leaves a time out, reset the timer and let her know there is no play until it runs its course, if possible without chasing them, screaming, or allowing the situation to unravel.

Without escalation, stick to your decision—don't interact, don't join in discussion, and don't lecture. Redirect them to the stairs, or wherever you have chosen, and start over again. Once children realize the ground rules, resistance usually stops, but when they've instead learned that time outs are up for debate, they'll debate.

TIME OUT BASICS

- Pick a spot, like a chair or a stair, away from social interactions or entertainment. Time outs need to be boring, away from the fun, with no play and no entertainment until they end. When sent to their room, children distract themselves with toys and forget they are in time out at all.
- Before giving a time out, if you'd like, offer your child one chance, without discussion, to correct their behavior: I'm going to count to three, and then you will get a time out.
- A general guideline for time outs is one minute per year of age, starting near two years.
- Stay calm. The punishment is the time alone, that's all.

- It can be a confusing concept—in essence we are saying some children have attention deficit hyperactivity disorder, but without the hyperactivity.

If your child is too active and impulsive to sit for a full one minute per year of age, they won't. Your expectations of how long a time out may need to change. But you require some way to enforce discipline in the house, and time outs avoid yelling, spanking, and other less-appropriate means. The length of time is not the critical piece; it is the removal of your attention.

Also avoid long lectures when discussing misbehavior. *How could you speak to me like that, we've given you everything, we try to give you responsibility but you don't hold up your end of the bargain, how would you like it if someone treated you like that...* These types of responses don't enforce the behavior you're looking for. A response needs to be immediate or it no longer connects with the actual event; children need to be able to connect the cause to the effect of their actions right away.

A discussion with a child is not a consequence. You don't often change behavior with logic, as young kids with ADHD are not particularly logical when planning their actions. They probably know why you felt their behavior was wrong, and they disagree. Or they messed up but without forethought—it was impulsive, a momentary distraction. As well, allowing a debate to continue too long also can lead to emotional escalation, a cyclical battle with no end.

Describing *why* they should behave differently still can be a long-term teaching tool. When you explain why your child should treat people well, or why a particular behavior is rude, you help them understand the abstract concepts of ethics and decorum even if it won't usually modify or teach behavior in the short run. Review these teaching points later, away from the acute conflict.

As always, a measure of balance is important. You do not want to create an impression that you are infallible and that children are powerless in your home. When not in the midst of managing behavioral issues, encourage children to express their opinions, and to collaborate in problem solving. Offer choices when you can but when a clear boundary has been crossed, discussion has to stop.

Aim to model calm, dispassionate discipline. "I'm sorry, but I counted to three and you didn't follow my directions, you are getting a time out." Or maybe instead, "Your video games are in time out the rest of the night." There's no need to engage or discuss beyond that. Some people worry time outs can come across as withholding affection, but the message is, "I love you and I want to play with you and I'm here for you, and you still cannot act like that."

8. Know Your Child

Your child has ADHD, a biological condition that affects self-regulation, memory, and everything else we've reviewed. Positive reinforcement, behavioral reward systems, and consistent limits, no matter how motivating, cannot undo their biology.

If your child hardly ever remembers to bring their homework home from school, motivation may not change that. They need a system of reminders, and to be taught a coping mechanism. They are forgetful because they are forgetful, it's the way their brain works and they need help.

Likewise, if a child is emotionally explosive, you might be able to work on a system to limit what happens when something triggers an out-of-control tantrum, like "no hitting." But you're not going to shut off the rage all together. In the short term even "no hitting" may be out of their control, and crisis management may involve creating a safe physical space in which to calm down.

On a related note, our society often treats teenagers as young adults when from a neurological point of view, they aren't. Again, the maturation of the frontal lobes into adulthood *begins* in teenagers, and reaches peak maturity in their twenties at the earliest. Before that happens, expecting a child to have a clear picture of the future, or a sense of long term consequences tied to their immediate behavior, or an understanding of why hard work makes you more successful down the road, may be unrealistic. They need adult guidance and supervision to learn and stay safe.

Collaborate and offer options when you can, remaining firm about some rules—such as use of the car—and lax when you feel comfortable. If there is some area of life you don't mind discussing and you're open to input, make it a collaborative decision—picking an after-school activity, choosing between two possible chores. Involve your child as much as possible while maintaining your perspective as a parent.

We're the grownups. We are the rational adults who reflect on our behavior and modify our responses. On a neurological level, we have mature frontal lobes and the capacity to plan for the future, and to learn from our mistakes. Parents influence children's behavior—that's why children need parents.

9. Maintain Perspective

Problem behaviors in children with ADHD are remarkably persistent. A child hits, they get a time out. They hit again, they get a time out. Forty times later you wonder what they are possibly thinking—but that's the point, without mature frontal lobes they are not thinking. Behavioral change requires an amazing amount of consistency and patience. If you set up a plan and expect results in a week, maybe you'll get lucky. But if that is your only measure of success, you may let yourself down. There will be steps forward and backward along the way.

Your child may be really happy coming to your bed every night. Now you've decided: It's time for you to sleep on your own. There is going to be push-back, a short-term escalation of problems before your child settles into a new equilibrium.

Adjusting the rules leads to frustration. You don't want your children to be upset and you don't want them to cry. You want them to be happy and well-adjusted. But you've made a decision: Your child needs to sleep through the night in his own bed. You change the routine.

From a child's perspective, they may not put a lot of stock into this announcement. You have attempted to get them to sleep in their own bed, and then when they fussed, you allowed them to stay. Once you make a stand, they become frustrated, and that's okay.

Just because you say or do something that makes your child upset does not mean you have hurt them or done anything wrong. It's your job to look at the big picture, make wise choices, and teach them how to do the same as they grow. If you too often give in, not only does your behavioral planning become ineffective, but you miss a chance to teach the ability to delay gratification, independence, and frustration tolerance.

You can also balance an awareness of what is inherent to a child's ADHD, at least for now, with what you can influence through your own actions. Kids with ADHD learn life skills more slowly than other children. They need repetition twenty or thirty times when other kids learn in three or four. They require a continued focus on routines, positive feedback, reward systems, and limit-setting. You'll need to maintain all of this in some manner pretty much until they leave home as young adults.

Lastly, we also want to avoid labeling everything related to ADHD as pathological. There's often a balance in knowing when to intervene and when to stand back. Some traits related to ADHD persist, but they don't impair life. After years of tension, it can be difficult to notice all the nuances of growth and progress. Where several years ago your child's exuberance wreaked havoc in the classroom, maybe now he's not disruptive. He's simply extroverted and a natural performer.

Finding a New Family Path

My daughter keeps calling me ever since my grandson Richard started treatment for ADHD. Richard cleared the table when she asked—without a complaint. He did his homework without fighting, the first time she asked. Suddenly, his teacher is sending home notes with stickers and stars almost every day. Until Richard started treatment, I don't think my daughter knew life could be any different. It's like a miracle has happened in their home.

⚜

Parenting influences ADHD but does not change its biology. Just because you want someone with an attention problem to respond quickly when you call doesn't mean they can. Intent on an art project, they aren't going to hear what you say. It's your job as a parent to adjust what you ask, how you ask, and your expectations. You cannot expect anyone to function in life at a higher level than their skills allow.

As with many medical conditions, symptoms rarely disappear through behavioral intervention alone. Expecting otherwise may increase your frustration level, and your child's. Major symptoms of ADHD, such as impulsivity, distractibility, or a struggle to complete activities, are generally affected more by medications, so we'll review both the safety and effectiveness of these options later in this section.

You'd like to say to your child, go clean up your room, and watch it happen. That doesn't mean they are physically capable of maintaining effort for long enough to finish, or to stay focused, or to avoid distractions. You may need to supervise, or create a poster to remind them of their chores, or help them organize the task, and the fact that these are needed may be immensely frustrating for you, as well as for them.

Some of these skills are taught over time. *You spend fifteen minutes before bed cleaning up, that's our family routine.* Eventually it even becomes habit, not discussed anymore. But attention shifting? That may not change much, and it may become your task to find a way to let go of habits and expectations. Shouting up the stairs to a child engrossed in their favorite TV show may not be an effective way of communicating when someone has ADHD.

A father once said to me, "It doesn't seem right. How small can I break down a task? I can't say, 'Go to the fridge. Put your hand on the handle. Open the door. Get out the milk. Pour the milk in the glass.' It isn't realistic. I can't live my life breaking down tasks like that all day long."

Hopefully your child can finish a task like pouring a glass of milk. But who can say? What is their memory like? How distractible are they? In fact, you may have to break down things like that for a while. What's important is, right now, can they complete this activity on their own, or can't they?

Here you are, problem solving. Your child for some unknown reason cannot get themselves a glass of milk properly and you've decided they need this life skill right away. Day after day milk leads to an explosive blow-up—mom or dad yelling and screaming, *You know better, we've told you what to do, you can do this on your own.*

And has that changed anything so far? The problem continues because they have ADHD, so they plan poorly, don't monitor their own behavior well, and are impulsive. They don't seem motivated to change that particular behavior, and maybe they like watching you pour their glass of milk.

Under stress, the potential responses we have to a situation dwindle. There may feel like there is this one answer: They have to try harder, this is not acceptable. You've tried reward systems when they were younger and now assume they'll never work. But they're older now. Maybe they're taking medication. Maybe they're working with a therapist, or maybe you are.

Could you structure the plan differently this time around? Are you consistent throughout the day in your limit-setting? Did you use your last plan for long enough? Could you ask someone outside the family for help?

You won't make the ideal choice every time. We all forget ourselves, or become overwhelmed, or get pushed too far at times. And sometimes we don't see a great way to handle something, and we pick whatever seems familiar, or whatever is the least unappealing option. This doesn't mean you've ever done anything right or wrong.

There is no perfect answer or perfect response. It is impossible to be calm and skillful in everything we do, all the time. But by remaining flexible to new possibilities for ourselves and for our children, our next choice may be the one that guides us into a new, less stressful future.

ANOTHER POINT OF VIEW

Picture a challenging interaction in detail, any recent situation that triggered your stress or felt as if it went awry. Imagining this conversation unfolding again, how does it make you feel physically? How do you hold your body, and what language and tone of voice do you use? How clearly do you think, and where do your thoughts go? What's your emotional state, and how does that affect what you say and do?[3]

Now pause. If the person you most respect in the world came into the room to handle this challenging situation for you, how would they act? Imagine this other person magically switched with you, no one else in the room knows they are even there. How would this change how you speak? What tone of voice would you now use? What would you say and do? If some phrase or emotional state (wisdom, compassion, calm) comes to mind, write it down as a reminder to yourself.

As you next enter a challenging situation, listen…pause… choose a response. Come back to your image, some sense of your intentions. What would be your most skillful reply, right now? If what you select turns out to be less than effective, that's fine. Reflect, plan to try something different the next time, or ask for advice if you need it.

Considering Therapy

It's hard for me. When I screwed up, my parents yelled or hit me. But with Robert, I'm trying to be different. I see that the calmer I stay, the calmer he stays. As angry as I feel, if I start shouting, he escalates too. If I'm quiet and stick to the plan, he's so much more compliant, and recovers quicker.

෴

When you find an inner voice nagging—*you should be able handle this,* or *if only my daughter would just be quiet and listen to me*—try to notice it as a thought and let it go. No one should judge you when you ask for help—least of all yourself. Instead of circling the wagons and shutting out the world, or losing yourself in a morass of conflicting advice from friends and neighbors, seek out someone with whom you can create a worthwhile plan of action.

When beginning with a therapist, a clear sense of your goals helps define what type of intervention will be most effective, or if therapy is likely to help at all. In general, clinical time spent working with parents influences a child's ADHD symptoms, and oppositional behaviors can be addressed along with adaptations for executive function problems. Therapy also can help parents begin to feel more in control of their family life. Individual therapy for a child is most effective for issues that go hand-in-hand with ADHD, such as low self-esteem and anxiety.

Make certain you are included in the process from the start. If months pass without any sense on your end of what's changing, ask the counselor to review with you the goals he set for you and for your child. Therapy with older children may require that they have additional confidentiality with the therapist, but even here parents should have some sense of the overall picture. To allow for this privacy, you may want to work separately with another therapist.

Managing Media: Let the Research Be Your TV Guide

Children with ADHD are at risk for a variety of related issues, including aggressive behaviors, poor eating habits, early experimentation with alcohol and sex, and a decreased ability to delay gratification. Television and other electronic media increase the risk of the exact same list. With ADHD in the house, media requires even closer monitoring than in other homes.

Don't underestimate the ill effects of media. Television, computers, video games, and other electronics are generally not a problem if well managed—but the research isn't subtle. They are, without a vigilant parent setting clear rules, bad for children. One of the most influential steps you can take as a parent is to implement appropriate media limits in your household.

Media, from television shows to computer games, functions as a useful diversion. Occasionally using a TV show so you can cook or get things done—not a problem. Television and video games entertain, and most of us have our favorite shows or watch sports or movies. But they also can take over a child's free time; one recent study showed that teens are spending roughly *all* of their waking life connected to some form of electronic media.[4]

Media has a profound influence on child development and there are benefits to limiting its use. For example, increased television hours correlate with an increased likelihood of aggressive behaviors. One study showed a decrease in aggressive behaviors after television hours were limited, even though the study did not specifically ask people to limit violent shows.[5] Another study showed a drop in academic performance over several months after video games were introduced into homes.[6]

Media time also increases the risks for obesity, alcohol use, and smoking.[7] Screen time replaces active play time and influences food choices. In younger children, background television may disrupt language development.[8] As children grow older, those who watch more television are more likely to start drinking and experimenting with sex earlier, and to try smoking. A 2010 study suggested television viewing at a young age increases the likelihood of sedentary behaviors, a preference for sugary snacks over fruits and vegetables, academic difficulty, and peer rejection.[9]

Advertising works. If it didn't work, millions of dollars would not be spent on it every day. Marketers carefully track the effectiveness of their commercials and refine them to make certain they have the most influence possible. Children and adults prefer products to which they have been exposed, and advertising generally does not push products that are healthy or worthwhile for children.

A DIFFERENT KIND OF TIME OUT

Every once in a while winter storms will shut down power to local towns for several days at a time. Families find themselves eating dinner together, playing games, and reading books side by side on the couch instead of separately watching television or sitting at the computer. Chatter follows in the community, and in my practice, about the bonding and warmth of the experience.

Why should we wait for Mother Nature? Periodically step outside the routines that have developed in your family, observe them, and set guidelines that promote your values. Maybe you'd like to pick a night each week, or even a block of time every night, to shut off electronics entirely. Try it for a month or two, and see what happens.

Media-driven culture encourages a short attention span and impulsivity, and the desire to have everything and buy everything right now. Yet an ability to delay gratification makes it more likely that children will succeed academically, socially, and behaviorally. In our homes, in our cars, on our children's phones, rapid-fire content assails our minds, rarely requiring more than a few minutes of sustained attention. Studies have correlated increased television time with a shorter attention span in children.[10] While far from proof that media causes attention problems, the theory makes sense. Allowing ourselves and our children to live under the barrage almost certainly affects brain development.

Media is not inherently "bad." Any individual child can thrive in any situation, and some children immersed in media will have no problems. But don't let media habits just happen to your family, consider them carefully. Make proactive, wise choices in your household—and notice what you model yourself.

Without isolating ourselves from the world, we can take steps to manage and corral media. There is no reason to think that kids will regulate their own time. In fact, children and teens with ADHD may be even more drawn to electronics and the Internet. Studies show the risk of Internet addiction is higher among teens and adults with ADHD.[11] Children require clear guidelines and limit-setting from their parents about television, computer, texting, and any other electronic connections right up to the time they move out of the house.

Guidelines for Media Use

Create clear rules. The American Academy of Pediatrics recommends two hours or less of combined screen time each day. Some families allow no media on school days, others none until homework is done. Avoid putting television sets in bedrooms and try to keep computers in public areas of the house. Most important to consider, however, is that children will not govern themselves—you must decide.

Choose the content. Even shows and games marketed to young children can contain inappropriate and violent content. Over the last generation, violence in cartoons has increased greatly, and the style of violence has become more realistic. Don't allow unsupervised web or channel surfing. Set up computers to limit access to content on the web, and allow visits only on websites with screened content. The industry standards are not developmentally appropriate. Check out content on your own, or use sites like www.commonsensemedia.org.

Avoid commercials. Use videos or digital recorders to minimize exposure to commercial content. If commercials didn't actually influence behavior, they wouldn't exist.

Avoid background television. If no one is watching a television, turn it off. Background television allows children to graze all day long, often with content that has shifted away from the program you selected. In addition, background television interferes with social interactions.

Model what you want your children to live. Emphasize family time over television time. Sitting side by side not interacting is not the same as actively playing together. Again, watching movies together is fun but needs to take its proper place in family life. Schedule family meals without setting a seat for television or computers. Beyond the benefits of regular family time, consistent family meals correlate with decreased rates of obesity in children and fewer high-risk behaviors in teens.

Set rules about other social media. Cellphones are beginning to cross into the world of "media," as newer models are more mini-computer than traditional phone. We do not know the social and developmental implications of over-using activities like texting, but there is nothing healthy about the social pressure to be always available, always part of the moment-to-moment gossip and banter. As well, the goal of being a teenager is to become a mature adult and constant contact with friends or parents through texting does not encourage independence. Without isolating your children from their peers, set clear limits. No electronics during meals or after a certain hour at night is a start.

The volume of texting and communication with peers often becomes excessive. There is no reason anyone, short of an emergency, needs to be texting during family time, games, or actual face-to-face time with another person. While these social boundaries have loosened, at a minimum treat the phone like a person intruding on conversation. Pause, politely excuse yourself, then check it if you must. *This could be an emergency, let me see who is calling.* And of course until the country catches up with clear laws, forbid your teens to text and talk on the cellphone when driving.

Establish safe use of the Internet. From an early age discuss and instruct in safe media use. While teens often know work-arounds, have someone set up programs on your computers that prevent unprotected Internet exploration. Monitor total hours and filter web content.

Teens aren't thinking of their future much of the time. They are impulsive to begin with—with ADHD, even more so. At an early age, remind children to treat anything they e-mail, text, or video as if it might be shared with the world. An innocent comment to a classmate—*I wonder if she likes me*—can become a tool of abuse for bullies when forwarded to an entire school.

No, I Will Not!

Forty percent or more of children with ADHD also have significant oppositional behavior, defined by defiant behaviors that persist at any given age beyond what is typical.[12]

Sometimes oppositional behaviors stem from ADHD alone—the emotional reactivity inherent to the condition. We all get frustrated throughout the day, but with ADHD there may not be a filter, leading kids to get upset or rattled and react without pausing. Other children may have a true "oppositional disorder," an inherent trait separate from their ADHD.

While there are many approaches to managing these behaviors, one of the better-known methods is that of Dr. Russell Barkley. His approach, available in books such as *Taking Charge of ADHD* and *Your Defiant Child,* begins with an emphasis on reestablishing a positive relationship with your child. It moves on to more traditional behavioral modification techniques, such as looking at the way parents make requests, and their use of rewards and consequences such as time-outs.

This structured, traditional behavior management approach parallels mindfulness training. As in a mindfulness class, Dr. Barkley asks parents to find positive experiences with their children and then make certain their children hear some acknowledgment of the behavior. In the midst of chaos, he asks that parents spend time each day with their children—simple enough, yet often hard to schedule and maintain. He asks for an objective look at a child's skills, and flexible problem solving.

But change is hard. We have our ways, tendencies to be too strict or too lenient, to ruminate on a single problem or to flit between issues without resolving any. Mindfulness training engenders a refocusing on positive interactions, an openness to new solutions, and compassion in understanding what it means to live with ADHD. Below is a framework for managing oppositional behaviors, integrating tools from both programs.

A related technique with problem behaviors, often referred to as the "ABC" approach, breaks them down into antecedent (what triggers the behavior), behavior (what actually happens), and consequences (the result). Any specific behavior has an underlying cause, and modifying a specific problem behavior begins by examining its function in more detail. Sometimes an action might be appropriate, like getting something to eat when hungry, and sometimes less so, like shoving a peer because you do not want to share toys. Sometimes a behavior may be biologically driven—I'm fidgeting because I have ADHD and cannot sit still, as my frontal lobes are not adequately supervising my motor activity.

You start by noticing what precedes the problem. Does the behavior always occur in a certain situation, such as transitioning from one activity to the next, or during unstructured time at recess? Is one particular child always involved, or does it happen at a particular time of day?

If you keep track of behaviors over a stretch of time, a pattern may emerge. Noticing the common causes of the behavior you've observed may allow proactive planning, anticipating, and heading off the problem before it happens. We need to supervise more when they play with Joey, or give them time to crash after school before starting school work. It also sometimes creates the option of avoiding a situation entirely for a while—maybe going to crowded stores isn't manageable right now.

Next you observe the behavior itself. If a child with ADHD has a temper, can you teach an alternative to lashing out? Or are those skills out of their control right now? Sometimes a straightforward alternative can be offered to replace the problem behavior—you cannot play with your brother's laptop, but I'll let you use mine with supervision.

By clarifying the results of a behavior, discipline often becomes clearer. Consequences of a behavior may be positive or negative for a child. If they push someone and get their toy, a child may see pushing as a positive. You may find yourself shouting and arguing because they do not want to start their homework. Your disapproval may seem like a negative, but the actual result your child got was exactly what he wanted—while you were talking, he was not doing his homework.

Guidelines for Oppositional Behaviors

Practice the skill of noticing yourself lost in mental distraction.
Return your attention to your actual experience, moment by moment,

hour by hour, and day by day. Notice when you're off in thoughts, plans, or ruminations over the past, or when you remain mentally enmeshed in a recent situation. At dinner, if you're still annoyed about how the morning went, you're going to miss the fact that your child has moved on and wants to hang out.

Focus your attention on your actual experience with your children. Most days, some small experience that is pleasant and enjoyable will happen. Some moments may be challenging, but many are not. Enjoy them, and make sure to focus your attention on the experience, and on your child, throughout. If there is a successful behavior to praise, praise it before anything else has happened.

Create time for your child each day. Whatever it takes, carve out some time daily for your child. Let them pick the activity, and follow their lead as much as possible. If you have more than one child you may need to alternate days, allowing each child to get your full attention for however much time you can reasonably carve out.

If your schedule seems too full for this, reevaluate your schedule. How are you spending your time? How much time on e-mail, television, Internet? Are there household responsibilities that can shift or can wait until after your child's bedtime, or the next day?

Monitor your own behavior. Monitor your own habits and emotional reactions around behavior management. If you escalate and yell or spank a child, you temporarily gain control but simultaneously teach that the loudest voice, or the heaviest hand, wins a confrontation.

But don't hold yourself to an impossible standard. You're going to lose your control at some point or another. Look with objectivity and compassion at what you tried, and don't give yourself a hard time. You did your best, but habits will crop up, again and again. Set out a new intention for the next time if you like. And then through steady practice and familiarity, you recover and move on sooner than before.

When you feel yourself agitated or overwhelmed, pause and focus on several breaths. Return your attention to the acute reality of the situation—and then choose a response. We often find our way out of habits when we draw our attention to them, so stop, take a measure of the situation, and then move forward.

Practice pausing before making requests. What do you anticipate asking? What do you really want to happen? Would it be possible to offer it as a choice—do you want dinner now or in fifteen minutes? Is your request important, or could you let it slide? Notice how you are holding yourself, and imagine the tone of voice you would like to use.

Notice what happens after you make a request. What is your child's response? How much does it mirror your behavior? Listen and pause, and find where you can agree while still maintaining your perspective as a parent. When you make a request, is it consistently followed? When you ask for something, be prepared to enforce it. Children are smart—if they learn that by pushing back they'll get their way, why should they stop pushing?

Begin behavior modification by emphasizing appropriate behaviors. As we noted earlier, start by noticing and praising the specific behaviors you want to promote. Then, create reward plans that reward the opposite of problem behaviors. Not only young children respond; a teenager can have his compliance increased around homework (or anything else) when earning something useful. Even when you are facing extreme behavioral challenges, select rewards that motivate, but then can be repeated over time.

Consistently uphold limits and rules. As noted earlier in this chapter, consequences are most effective when they are immediate and do not escalate the situation. In the midst of enforcing discipline, there is little point in discussion. That can wait until later. Right now, engaging in a circular debate when you've already decided to enforce a rule only lets the situation build. Consequences may include time outs or temporary loss of certain toys or privileges, such as television or video game time.

When a behavioral plan isn't working, reexamine the plan. Does your plan account for your child's true abilities, right now? One common reason systems fail is that a child just doesn't have the skill yet. If they are fundamentally impulsive, you won't accomplish enough by emphasizing the rules *(don't hit)* without offering alternative skills through other behavioral or medical interventions. The bar needs to be set slightly above their present skill level, with a goal of more success than failure. As well, remember to maintain focus on incremental progress, as change happens slowly.

Seek expert help. When oppositional behaviors occur in a child with ADHD, try your best, but always remember: You're a parent, not a behavioral management super-genius. Maybe you've read a book that felt useful, but you still don't have a handle on everything. That's entirely to be expected. These situations are immensely complex and clinicians complete years of training to understand them. When you feel stuck, reach out to someone with the clinical background to help.

KEEP IT MOVING

Build your mental strength and flexibility as you might approach a physical work out. Not everyone enjoys the same kind of physical exercise. Luckily, we can choose from hiking, jogging, biking, dance, weight training, yoga, and endless other options. Likewise, meditation does not have to be about sitting still. Traditionally, it has been guided sitting, standing, lying down, and walking, and what's most natural for one person may frustrate another.

Yoga is a form of meditation, as are various martial arts, like tai chi. While it is a form of physical exercise, yoga also cultivates mindfulness and focused awareness of the body. Poses are meant for exploration, as not everyone fits some kind of physical ideal. Movements and exercises can be modified, and where one person glides into a split, another stretches their back a few gentle degrees forward. One pose is no better or worse than the other, with each person exploring their own limit.

Walking meditation exists in many formats. One style can be practiced almost anywhere. Walking naturally, focus your attention on the experiences around you, as you do with your breath. Eyes open, notice sounds and smells, the sensation of lifting your legs and placing them on the ground, and whatever comes into your field of vision. Walk at a natural pace, unforced, observing the world around you.

This style of meditation works anywhere. In the middle of a city street, rushing from one meeting to the next, focus on the chaos. All the noise and honking horns and people rushing and shouting—practice observing it all without harsh reactions or judgments. Take care of yourself along the way, avoiding dangers, stopping at corners. Maintain a balanced awareness of everything going on.

Walking meditation can also be guided in a more structured fashion. Choose a location, indoors or out, where you're able to walk five or ten paces, and then pay more direct attention to each aspect of taking a step. The lifting of your foot, the shift of weight that occurs simultaneously, the sensation of your muscles and joints moving as you swing your leg forward, and then placing your foot again on the ground. Walk at your typical pace if you'd like, or slow down to a measured pace, making each movement with intention. Pause at your turning point, and wait to make your turn until the moment you choose.

As always, none of these choices are better or worse than any other. If walking feels easier for you than sitting, then walk. Perhaps notice where the challenge is with sitting meditation, and return to it some other time. Choose yoga if you'd like. Find whatever fits for you, and dedicate yourself to a consistent practice.

CHAPTER 8

Education: Rallying the Team

*U*nderstanding ADHD and knowing the educational options available help you advocate for your child. Parents often need to guide schools toward various classroom supports, academic accommodations, and curriculum choices. Children also benefit when teachers understand ADHD neurobiology. Getting off task, not listening when called, speaking out of turn in class, being forgetful, having emotional outbursts, and endless other ADHD-related problems in school again trace back to poor frontal lobe function. These ADHD-driven challenges call for short-term supports along with long-term planning that builds skills and offers strategies to compensate.

❧

Revisit the Brain Manager

He's failing two classes again. The teacher keeps telling me he isn't handing in his homework. I go through his bag and there are blank worksheets. He thinks they might be work he didn't finish in class, but he says he doesn't remember. I have no way of knowing. There's a missing piece of communication somewhere. Who am I supposed to ask?

❧

For most children, school requires more executive function skills than other parts of their life. For starters, they must control their activity level enough to sit still, and they must deal with their impulses while listening and waiting their turn. They need to focus on their teacher, blocking out distractions in the room—as well as internal distractions, like thoughts of the new toy waiting at home. They must find the ability to organize and process what they've heard, as well as to retrieve it, paraphrase it, and get it down on paper. And then as they get older, they are expected to keep track of assignments and books independently, manage their time, and plan ahead. It is no wonder many people in the field consider executive function deficits to be a learning disability on their own.

When ADHD is first identified, planning often focuses on behavior management at school and at home. Initial interventions may be directed at impulsivity, fidgeting, daydreaming, and class disruptions. Children, especially those with hyperactivity or impulsivity, must be able to sit, focus, and control their impulses enough to participate. They need to interact with peers and teachers appropriately. And then there are the equally pressing and less obvious issues such as scattered organizational skills, poor time management, and working memory deficits. Again, it's not only the most obtrusive ADHD symptoms that matter.

ADHD isn't an excuse for school problems or misbehavior, but it can be an explanation. Children with ADHD do not know how to keep track of their work, organize their time, or maintain effort. The overriding question should never be *Why don't they work harder?* but, *Since they don't have this skill yet, what can we do to help?*

Many common ADHD symptoms in the classroom are cataloged on the initial diagnostic checklist (page 27): Trouble with focus, impulsively speaking out of turn, fidgeting, hyperactivity, and all the rest. A careful observation may find troubles in many of the areas listed below as well, and this is only a partial list:

- Keeping track of a day planner without misplacing it.
- Keeping track of paperwork and handing it in appropriately.
- Maintaining a written to-do list, holding on to mental instructions or lists.
- Organizing and maintaining a book bag, locker, or desk.
- Organizing thoughts for narrative writing.
- Planning projects and anticipating time.
- Reading and remembering instructions.

- Identifying problems, checking for errors, and learning from mistakes.
- Transitioning between activities and starting new activities.

Optimal school planning therefore includes a meticulous look at executive function. Does your child know how to look at the board, write an assignment down in the appropriate place, get their assignment pad into the backpack, get their backpack home, find their assignment list, and get started on homework? Or are they lost at the first step? Can they sit for a test, read the instructions without missing details, maintain focus, remember the instructions three questions later, and do all of that without making careless errors?

Allowing children with executive function struggles to bang their head against an academic wall over and over again undermines motivation. If they knew how to figure it out on their own, they would, and children with ADHD may give up academically without outside help. Though distractible, impulsive, or poorly organized, they may know what they are supposed to be doing in class. When they fail anyway, they eventually stop trying. It's human nature. To avoid this situation, we must build academic skills and motivation through an emphasis on each small step along the way, guiding children to the point that they have the knowledge, skills, and confidence needed to continue on their own.

To create true academic motivation, children must feel a sense of control and experience both mastery of a skill set and success. Children rarely maintain inspiration created out of fear—*do your homework or else I'll take away your video game.* In the short term, alarm over an impending loss gets the job done; long-term drive doesn't follow. Intensive supports that prevent falling behind must be coupled with instruction in skills that promote independence. Children are taught what to do to keep up in school, and then repeat those skills until they are mastered, enabling a child to shift from keeping up to excelling.

Executive function interventions at school apply equally at home. You create a short-term safety net: These are the areas in which my child is having difficulty, and right now their abilities are at this stage of their development. You balance this with a long-term plan: How can we best build new proficiencies and create systems to compensate for ADHD, while maintaining a clear goal of independence and success? While you cannot dictate every moment of your child's day at school, familiarizing yourself with teaching techniques effective for ADHD strengthens your ability as an advocate.

The Whole Academic Picture

Children with ADHD may fall behind solely because of ADHD-related symptoms. They miss out on instruction while distracted, daydreaming and off task. Over years, the gap may grow large. Prolonged catch-up may be required because hundreds of hours have been lost and information missed.

ADHD directly causes academic problems as well. When reading, children with ADHD often miss word endings, small words, and modifiers, or skip lines entirely, little pieces of information that nuance stories. Working memory is also critical for reading because as children read, they must hold onto information from the beginning to the end of a line, or a paragraph, or a story. By the end of a passage, kids with ADHD have lost track of the start, an error that affects comprehension. You cannot understand what you are reading if you miss these details.

While skilled reading appears effortless, learning to read is work. Reading is hard for many kids with ADHD, and distractibility and poor focus are exacerbated by any task that isn't highly engaging. Because of this, kids with ADHD often don't like reading books, starting a vicious cycle. Reading fluency builds from reading practice, yet ADHD may push children away from books, further limiting their progress and making the task even more difficult and distasteful over time.

Similarly, math skills lag in many children with ADHD. Completing problems efficiently, and getting to the correct answer, depends on paying attention to the details and mental manipulation of facts, which requires working memory. ADHD also impairs a child's ability to self-monitor and leads to rushing, so there may be frequent careless mistakes.

Writing is one of the hardest academic skills for students, requiring both a knowledge base and a host of executive function skills to synthesize a coherent composition. ADHD affects the ability to retrieve information, organize thoughts, and get it all written down in a linear and well-formed fashion. Direct teaching of skills such as how to organize ideas in an outline, compose a draft, and edit toward a final version is needed, and often underemphasized in schools today.

While children with ADHD require extra help because of all of their ADHD-related problems, you still cannot assume ADHD causes every issue. Up to half, if not more, of children with ADHD have a related learning disability, hard-wired deficits with acquiring an academic skill.[1] Children with ADHD are at risk for disorders in areas such as reading, math, and narrative writing, all of which benefit from targeted, skill-based teaching from the start.

The frontal lobes—everything comes back to this brain region in ADHD—supervise aspects of motor control. This can relate to handwriting, leading to a condition called dysgraphia in some. Children with ADHD often have difficulty with motor control, which can cause a "developmental coordination disorder." To determine if any of these learning disabilities are present, detailed educational testing may be pursued as soon as academic issues become apparent, and becomes mandatory when academic problems persist.

❧

Teaching is an art that, like parenting, should be guided by science. In many ways, however, the true craft is in the application of the science. For all areas of academics, and for any child at risk academically, there are evidence-based methods of teaching that increase the odds of success. Although each child needs a unique approach and individualized attention, decades of educational research inform teachers in their instructional choices and you can further advocate for your child by requesting appropriate programs. Students with ADHD should be offered highly structured curricula based on scientific research. Programs include:

- A beginning reading program strong in phonics that includes reading aloud with a teacher.
- A math program that teaches basic math facts and algorithms.
- A writing program that stresses outlining and planning to help students organize thoughts and stay on topic.
- Individualized instruction in organizational skills such as note-taking, time management, and test-taking.[2]

Through exposure to these methods, learning problems can be minimized. Academics should be presented through direct instruction in a well-organized classroom. Direct instruction emphasizes working in small groups composed of students at similar skill levels, under the supervision of a teacher who provides continuous reinforcement and correction. A well-organized classroom ensures there is a clearly delineated front of the room with students facing forward. Visual clutter and noise should be kept to a minimum.

For reading instruction, programs that emphasize a systematic cultivation of targeted skills minimize the likelihood any child will fall behind. A far higher percentage of children thrive when schools use structured, evidence-based approaches to reading than with other methods. Children benefit from programs that follow guidelines such as those put forth by the National Reading Panel in 2000.[3]

Current approaches to math often emphasize the process of figuring out problems more than fluency in basic math facts. Again, math proficiency more likely follows from traditional methods that build basic skills. A foundation of well-learned math facts facilitates the acquisition of higher-level skills.

Advocate for these teaching methods. Some children will thrive with any curriculum choice but many of those with ADHD struggle. They generally succeed with the sequential teaching methods reviewed above. If they are not used in your school district, seek a tutor.

Of course, there is never one cookie-cutter approach to teaching. We consider the percentages, recognizing that certain curricula meet the needs of more children than others. After that, education requires frequent reassessment followed by adjustments in instructional techniques. Regardless of the initial interventions utilized, the bottom-line measure for any child is nothing more than their own progress.

Know Your Rights

Parents have legal rights that make certain their child's academic needs are met. By federal law, school systems must evaluate children who are struggling and establish an appropriate plan to intervene. While schools can initiate the process, they are also required to evaluate children after parents make a written request.

As discussed in chapter two, school-based evaluators do not typically make medical diagnoses such as ADHD. Parents can, on their own, involve a developmental pediatrician, psychologist, neurologist, or psychiatrist at any time. These outside providers add their independent evaluation to school testing, help parents understand the schools results, and act as an advocate throughout the process.

Once evaluation is complete, a school decides if a child requires an individualized educational program (IEP), a 504 plan, or neither. Mandated by federal law, an IEP addresses specific conditions such as learning disabilities that require special education, therapies, or self-contained classes. A 504 plan (referring to section 504 of the Rehabilitation Act of 1974 and also called "504 accommodations") covers children who may need supports because of a disability (such as ADHD) but do not require special education services. These 504 plans do not have as strict legal requirements regarding their implementation or evaluation process as an IEP.

Schools sometimes implement academic plans without creating an official document based on the federal mandate. Since the ultimate goal of teachers and administrators is to meet the needs of each child, they may decide that a written plan is unnecessary to offer assistance. On a practical level this approach works as long as a child gets the help they need. However, an official plan is easier to monitor and allows continuity of the program when teachers or classrooms change.

For children with ADHD, a 504 plan is often the starting point because it calls for interventions implemented in a mainstream setting. All of the academic, organizational, and behavioral care outlined in this chapter can be initiated in this manner. Since schools often develop 504 accommodations without detailed educational testing to determine if learning disabilities or other academic-related issues are present, if children continue to struggle further evaluation should take place.

Children with passing grades still may require 504 services. Because of the executive function problems inherent to ADHD, students put in draining amounts of effort to compensate for forgetfulness, distractibility, disorganization, or an inability to manage time. School staff may not be aware of the amount of energy parents expend propping up homework and studying at home. Entering a planning meeting with a clear view of where your child is struggling and potential accommodations a school may offer will help you be certain he gets all the help he requires.

While many students with ADHD begin with a 504 plan, this intervention is not always sufficient. When children have significant learning, behavioral, or development concerns, or their ADHD alone causes them to require small group instruction, another level of educational intervention may be needed. These more intensive interventions or self-contained classrooms are available only through special education placement implemented through an IEP. If academic concerns persist after 504 services start, parents should request a full psychoeducational evaluation to enable the creation of an appropriate plan.

Communication with the School

Aim to make meetings between school personnel and families low-key, stress-free, with everyone working towards a shared goal. Strive to remain calm and knowledgeable. Staff and parents can collaborate to support each individual child, flexibly compromising when necessary, and plans can evolve over time based on a child's response. If you have a clear view of the services your child requires and are able to document why they are necessary, an appropriate solution eventually should be reached. While there may be differences of opinion and perspective, everyone involved is there to help your child progress.

Ongoing discussions with school personnel provide opportunities to practice quiet resolve. Sometimes the planning process does not feel collaborative, and the system can be confusing. You may want more for your child than a school feels is needed. Or, teachers may feel your child needs special help, but you don't. When there is a disagreement over what needs to be done, tensions often rise.

If an impasse is reached, parent advocates are available in most communities to support families, and parents can request their presence at school meetings. As a last resort, educational lawyers can be immensely helpful in defending the rights of individual children.

If the air begins to feel heavy, you can practice mindfulness. Calm yourself, stepping aside for a few moments to settle your thoughts. Even when you disagree with school officials, you might learn some useful piece of information when you attend quietly. You can practice again: Listen. Pause. Respond.

With resolution and strength, always advocate for your children. But practice mindfulness even in this potentially tense communication, pausing, listening, and responding with clarity and perspective. As often as needed, remind yourself that schools must always meet the needs of every child. Clear communication is the key to getting your child the help they require.

Be Open and Honest

There are instances in which parents do not tell the school about their child's ADHD. Yet teachers and school psychologist still know that there is a problem, and chatter follows children from classroom to classroom and grade to grade. This may compound the problem because the label exists, but without a targeted plan. Relationships between the school and parents often become strained. It's far better to work collaboratively on a solution than to bang heads with teachers or psychologists frustrated by a lack of parental support.

Parents are often concerned that a school will "label" their child with ADHD, or they worry that having the diagnosis on paper will taint or limit their experience. But without the diagnosis, the best-intended school plan will fall short. School personnel must recognize ADHD to know where to start. They also need the diagnosis to qualify a child for supports, as a specific finding is often required when creating a 504 or IEP.

By sharing an ADHD diagnosis with schools, you allow the school to take the steps needed to intervene. Children benefit when their teachers identify and attribute ADHD-related symptoms accurately. A comprehensive educational plan permits children to take control of their environment, and to master their academic world in a way that is not possible on their own.

Refining the Plan

Often what happens to parents at school meetings is that they face a whirlwind of information about all the possibilities and decisions that have already been made (we feel he does not need a 504 plan). They are given a checklist of what's going to be done (so we're giving him time-and-a-half on tests and preferential seating), and then leave utterly confused. They have little idea what their options are, both legally and in defining any of the details that could help their child at school. Unless involved with a clinician outside the system, they have no way of knowing if the plan is adequate or not.

Familiarizing yourself with the possibilities will help you guide your children through the system, so a broad compilation of possible educational intervention strategies is reviewed below. Effective educational interventions fall into several categories: behavioral plans, classroom and organizational help, homework, and testing supports. Of course, not every child needs every possible service or item on the list.

In reviewing what these supports entail, keep in mind that most of the details that follow will address teachers, not parents. Your awareness of them, however, allows you to make valuable observations and ask relevant questions. Don't hesitate to discuss additions to the school program if you think your child would benefit from them.

Behavioral Planning

Create a structured behavioral plan in the classroom before problems develop. Proactive use of behavioral plans has been shown to improve behavior in class and completion of work, decrease carelessness, and diminish other ADHD-related behavior problems.[4] Schools sometimes wait to see if a child is going to have problems in a new setting; you can instead ask them to establish a plan that emphasizes praise, reward, and expectations that account for a child's ADHD-related impairments from day one in the class, or for any new situation.

Review the plan with everyone involved. Make certain the behavioral plan includes clear rules, displayed in writing, and is tied to rewards instead of only punishment. Before tensions develop with your child, encourage a new teacher to follow the same basic guidelines reviewed in the last chapter. Some teachers may even choose to implement a program on a classroom-wide level, since many of the guidelines apply to all students.

The system should be similar to the one you use at home, if possible, including use of immediate consequences. One note for school planning is that recess and physical activity may be correlated with improved behavior in children with ADHD; cutting recess as a punishment can prove to be counter-productive.

Expectations should be similar across classrooms and, when possible, between home and school. Behavioral change comes quickest when all the adults involved follow the same consistent message. A "home report card" may detail behavioral goals and successes, and has been shown to reduce ADHD symptoms in school. This daily or weekly communication also allows parents and teachers to coordinate their planning and monitoring efficiently.

Request adaptations for more specific ADHD-related behaviors and problems. For example, kids with ADHD need reminders to stay on task more than their peers, so teachers can create subtle cues at the start of the school year: *If I tap your desk, I'm reminding you to get back on task*. Kids with ADHD require more repetition to learn, and follow directions. They benefit from visual cues and lists, unburdened by the expectation they will keep track of everything in their heads.

Monitor teacher expectations. Over time a child with ADHD may catch up to their peers, but in the short run they simply may not have the ability to sit in place, or focus consistently. Punishing someone because of a behavior they cannot control isn't a long-term solution. A child may fidget without disrupting class, or may get to take a break if he asks appropriately. Reasonable allowances can be made for any individual child if they do not disrupt rest of the classroom.

Anticipate and plan for problem situations. Most often, schools will create programs that anticipate and manage challenging parts of the day without your guidance. However, you also can make certain school staff are aware of specific situations in which your child would benefit from additional support. If transitions are always challenging, ask your child's teachers to create a routine that prepares them to shift activities. When that fails, teachers can emphasize reward systems. If a specific activity like recess is always a challenge, request that staff offer more supervision on the playground, or set up more structured activities for play. And if standard interventions fail, a psychologist or social worker in the school may be available to observe what's going on and create a special plan for your child.

Classroom and Organizational Supports

Monitor classroom structure. Chaotic, disorganized classrooms challenge children with ADHD. Distractions on the walls or from other unruly children aggravate symptoms. Inconsistent schedules cause confusion. And unstructured policies around school work, such as when it is done or handed in, muddle your child's budding systems for managing their day. When possible, encourage placement of your child with teachers who run more structured, consistent classrooms.

Preferential seating for children with special needs is not out of the ordinary. A child with ADHD usually does best when seated toward the front of the room, away from doorways and windows and away from individual children who cause distractions. Group seating, now used often as a standard seating arrangement instead of only for collaborative assignments, has been shown to exacerbate behavioral issues. For children with ADHD, sitting between two friends and across from three others adds another obstacle to learning.[5]

Monitor classroom placement and schedule. If your child is never able to manage their workload, talk to the school about adjusting their schedule. Children with ADHD are sometimes offered time during the day to receive adult support to organize school work or to catch up on specific subjects, in a setting often called a "resource room." More specific changes in a schedule, such as dropping a foreign language requirement, can help lower the overall workload. When academic or behavioral issues persist, consider getting your child into a smaller, special education setting. This may help minimize ADHD symptoms all on its own, by decreasing the ratio of students to teachers and allowing more direct academic instruction.

Remember attention management. Teachers can support children with short attention spans. Children can be allowed to get up and move at defined times. During prolonged stretches of intense work, teachers can anticipate the need for breaks, and schedule them. A teacher can let a child know they'll be working hard for fifteen minutes, then can stretch and get a drink of water and come back, setting realistic goals based on the performance they've seen.

Provide direct instruction in organizational skills. Organization and planning are chronic problems for ADHD students. Even as children outgrow more disruptive symptoms, these difficulties persist. They reflect a brain not yet ready to manage information smoothly.

For most students, the process of writing an assignment down in a day planner once a teacher puts it on the board becomes intuitive. But the expectation that a child with ADHD will look at the blackboard, remember to write down their homework on paper without missing any details, get the list home, and understand what he's written down, may not be as realistic. What seems like a simple task turns out to have multiple, challenging steps.

A short-term solution assigns an adult at school to monitor the day planner. There is often a "check out" at the end of the day to make certain kids have their books and a complete assignment list. Direct contact with parents regarding what is due for the week helps as well.

A long-term plan requires a structured, step-by-step program that builds independence. It balances learning new skills with promoting some measure of self-awareness and self-reliance. A child may never be instinctively neat or organized. So what habits can we teach?

Similarly, taking notes may be an epic hurdle in ADHD, often complicated by struggles with focus, working memory, and handwriting. Assistance with note-taking allows children to continue progressing with class content. These accommodations may include providing an outline, providing notes ahead of time, or permitting access to notes after class has ended. Direct instruction in note-taking should also be considered.

Help children manage time. The same part of the brain responsible for organization manages time. When it is underactive, estimating and managing time becomes a huge hurdle, so children with ADHD generally struggle with predicting how long an assignment will take. *I'll have it done in twenty minutes...* and three hours later, the task continues.

Initially, an adult guides children in breaking down longer-term projects to develop this new habit. The adult makes certain each step is recorded in the day planner as daily work. They can delineate the details of producing an essay, from picking a topic, researching, outlining, and writing all the way to proofreading. At home, you might allocate fifteen minutes for more general studying each day, encouraging long-term thinking about school work.

Testing, Testing

Rarely, a request for a 504 plan can be misguided—a parent asking for extended time for tests, seeking a competitive advantage. Of course, these aren't usually parents of children who actually have ADHD. But as it turns out, more time is not always a useful support for kids with ADHD.

It is true that a subgroup of kids with ADHD works slower than peers. They remain inefficient in their pacing and problem solving in spite of getting help and actually require extended test time for fair evaluation.

Equally common with ADHD are children who are distractible and get off task if their classmates are around. Or while testing, they miss instructions or skip lines or make careless errors. A more effective accommodation for these children, therefore, is moving them away from distractions. You also can ask to have someone make sure children read and follow the instructions.

As a companion to modifications, other testing skills can be taught directly. A teacher can show children how to reread and circle the pertinent parts of the question, or how to mark up salient features of a paragraph. Kids can learn to make a habit of rechecking answers, even if their instinct is to rush through. And expect that from the start, adult prompting and supervision will be required for a long, long time, creating another opportunity for parents and teachers to coordinate their actions.

Find out if grading can be adjusted for academic issues driven by executive function. Some children and teens cannot get ideas on paper for an essay test because of handwriting issues, for example, and may need to be able to type, or be scored on multiple choice—style questions to accurately gauge their knowledge. As well, kids who cannot yet adeptly organize an essay should not lose credit over and over again across all their classes because of this one skill. Overall assessments can be weighted to emphasize in-class work, homework, or whatever most accurately reflects a child's effort and knowledge.

Homework Support

To complete their homework students must have the skills to take their day planner home, pack their homework and the correct books, locate and open their day planner later, arrange their belongings, and assemble their thoughts. And then, of course, they must be capable of the organizational pirouette required to monitor themselves and stay focused until done, clean their desk, and place everything exactly back where it belongs in their book bag so it can be handed in the next day.

This organizational, motivational, and working memory dance defines ADHD. Each step involves an interaction of cognitive abilities including focus, planning, and persistence. Children with ADHD are delayed in developing these skills. For homework to smoothly function, you must define the initial routine until it becomes ingrained.

Your child's teacher may need to confirm everything is written down. A simple verbal reminder may not be enough, even though it suffices for other kids in class. The long-term goal is independence; the short-term step is an unbiased appraisal of a child's capacities, right now, today. It's up to parents to create set routines and boundaries around homework. Children with ADHD have a hard time recognizing when to start, how to stay on task, and how to plan their time. Close communication with teachers or other school staff regarding assignments and teacher expectations will be helpful as well. Here are basic guidelines for home:

Create a homework schedule. A consistent homework routine builds life skills. You might have a morning or bedtime plan that remains relatively fixed day to day, and you can do the same with homework. Every night you brush your teeth before bed and every day when you return from school, have a snack, and do your work, in that order.

Pick a time to start homework. Stick to it, varying for after-school activities as needed. Once it is routine, you often will find less arguing and resistance.

For families using ADHD medications, consider medication timing in planning homework. Homework will be more efficient and manageable when children are permitted the benefits of their medication. Starting homework after dinner or late at night is a return to unmedicated ADHD, so it may take much longer than if done earlier in the day. Share this concept with your kids, because eventually they will recognize that work takes thirty minutes with medication, one hour without.

Create a homework location. In order to permit adult supervision, children with ADHD often complete homework in central areas of the house, like the kitchen table. However, these areas are often full of distractions—people coming and going, cooking, phone calls, or television. Ideally, create an uncluttered, consistent space, away from the center of the house and away from toys.

Carve out a setting separated from media as much as possible. If computer use is needed, set a policy of turning off email and instant messaging while working. A household rule of no television or video games until homework is done may minimize distractions as well.

Use a homework checklist. Write down and post a step-by-step homework plan that will evolve over time. Common starting points on the list are:

- Take out your to-do list.
- Confirm you have information from every class—either assignment details or "no homework due."
- Check that you have all the materials you need.

- Start working.
- Check your work before leaving your desk.

Use a timer. Children often focus more easily when they know a break is coming, and also may work more effectively with short bursts of effort. Pick a time period of fifteen to thirty minutes, and set a timer. Monitor the breaks as well or they may extend indefinitely, setting aside five or ten minutes, preferably to stretch or use the bathroom, not to play.

As children grow older, these chunks of time can be used to learn time management. Older children can predict how long their work will take, and compare their prediction to their actual experience. You can begin to show them the difference between their perception and reality—every time you guess thirty minutes for writing, it takes an hour. You can also schedule future thinking: After today's work is done, schedule twenty minutes of study for something due later in the week.

Create a single homework folder. A chronic problem for children with ADHD is that homework, when it is done, gets left at home, in the backpack, or in the locker. Or vanishes entirely. It disappears into the same void as permission slips and school forms.

Choose a single, brightly colored folder, and encourage placing any completed papers in that folder only. Use the folder for nothing else, so that the moment anything is done, that's where it goes. Then build a habit with help from school staff of checking that the folder is empty at school. As long as the folder is clear at the end of the day, everything has been handed in.

Use reward systems to enhance motivation. Award points each day when work is completed appropriately and without complaint. After a certain number of points a small prize is earned—typically around a week's work for younger children, and up to a month or two for older ones.

Monitor homework time. Homework is not meant to be punitive. It is a tool for supporting classroom learning and building academic skills. However, it becomes counterproductive after a point. A general guideline is ten minutes per grade level (that is, thirty minutes total in third grade).

Homework is hard enough without the added stress of having it engulf entire nights, an issue which may be addressed by limiting the number of examples to complete. Likewise, if handwriting is a specific concern for your child and slows work, discuss using a keyboard or note-taking help. Don't hesitate to speak to your school about homework modifications when needed.

Hit the reset button. A child is barely getting by with studying and handing in most assignments…and then by November, they've also accumulated a pile of stuff that needs to be made up. What was close to manageable now involves not only the daily workload, but catching up. It can lead to a monumental shut-down. When productivity and motivation plummet it even may look like medications have stopped working. In reality, it's a skill-based issue, and the child doesn't know how to tackle the mess. They need someone to parse it out, perhaps to amend or release them from obligations, and help to put together a manageable plan.

SUMMARY OF ACADEMIC ACCOMMODATIONS FOR ADHD

While the potential list of accommodations is nearly endless, here are some of the most common to which you can refer:

- Seat the child toward the front of the room, away from distractions
- Consistently use structured behavioral plans
- Schedule breaks during class time
- Assist in writing down homework assignments
- Assist in keeping track of books and materials (including duplicate books at home if needed)
- Offer note-taking help, such as providing outlines (or even entire sets of notes in children who do not yet have the ability to take them)
- Break down longer assignments into smaller parts
- Extend test time for children who cannot finish on time or whose performance drops when under time pressure
- Test away from distractions
- Monitor to make certain test instructions are followed
- Modify homework (for example, limiting the number of items to be completed)
- Permit keyboard use for homework (instead of handwriting)
- Provide instruction in organizational skills
- Modify grading, such as emphasizing knowledge of content in essays until writing skills have developed

Adjust the Academic Plan Over Time

Nothing in life is static and unchanging. Children with ADHD will grow and learn new skills, perhaps requiring fewer supports in some areas. They mature and take more responsibility, allowing more freedom to create their own methods for managing their workload. But through the years academic demands escalate, and more supervision and care may be needed in upper grades.

Many children with ADHD stumble when they hit middle school. The requirement for independence takes a leap forward, and solid academic and executive function skills, from fluent reading abilities to ease with writing thought-out essays, are required. The number of transitions and long-term assignments grows and issues that were once manageable become overwhelming. A new level of impairment caused by ADHD becomes apparent, or perhaps the possibility of ADHD is raised for the first time.

The symptoms of ADHD also evolve over time. As they mature, some children cease to fidget, act impulsively, and daydream. But even when children no longer demonstrate the "by the books" checklist of ADHD symptoms, they often battle persistent executive function deficits.[6] If a child outgrows their ADHD diagnosis, or seems to be well-behaved and well-focused in the classroom, many of the supports you've fought for may be withdrawn. Sometimes this makes sense, as skills have matured and help is no longer needed. But challenges with self-regulation, planning, managing time, and completing work continue...and require continued, intensive supports throughout schooling.

EXPLORE YOUR MENTAL HABITS

Dealing with educational issues, from your child's chronic struggles to negotiating services with schools, triggers endless reactions, pushing the mind back onto its roller coaster. Here we go again. I'm frustrated, tired, anxious, angry, fearful...and your brain jumps onto the familiar ride, and then whips around the well-worn track.

As you practice letting the mind settle you start to become familiar with the places it wanders. You slow down and realize, here I am again, feeling rushed and sprinting through the morning. I've been here before, relieved and content. This is familiar—tired and angry. Once again now, ruminating.

Through meditation, you can familiarize yourself with these patterns, perhaps giving yourself an opportunity for change. Sit for several minutes, or as much time as you like, watching your breath. Start by noticing the sensations wherever most obvious to you, in your belly or chest, or the sensation of air moving.

Continue to use your breath as a place to return when distracted. And then begin to observe the emotions and thoughts as they come and go. At times they may be scattered and fast paced, as though you were standing in the midst of a raging storm. At times they may be thick and slow-moving like a fog.

Instead of focusing only on your breath, for a few minutes watch your emotional state. You may feel tired, bored, angry, relaxed, restless…or nothing in particular at all, just calm. For these few minutes, notice your feelings come and go, pleasant or unpleasant, without striving to do something, or change anything. You might briefly label what you feel—unhappy, ecstatic, quiet, irritable. And then again, return to the breath.

Even comfortable, pleasant emotional experiences can be sticky and lead to unrest. If you're relaxed and happy, notice that. Notice again any physical sensations in your body that arise, any thoughts or expectations or desires. Enjoy them. But recognize as well, everything comes and goes. If you expect meditation to be peaceful and easy, each and every time, you'll set yourself up for disappointment. Enjoy moments of relaxation and happiness as long as they last, without effort. When your experience or mood shifts, notice that change without resentment or frustration.

It's a common habit to push away from unpleasant experiences, to shut down, or feel an urge to get up and do something else. If you're able, notice how even uncomfortable feelings and emotions shift, ebbing and flowing over time. Notice any physical sensations that accompany these internal states. Practice sitting and for a few breaths not reacting, not doing anything at all.

Remember you can always take care of yourself. If you're overwhelmed, make an adjustment. Open your eyes. Sometimes through observation, a feeling or sensation does change—and other times it remains uncomfortable and we find it best to move our attention away.

When you're ready, shift your attention to your thoughts. You might begin to notice, over time, the ruts your mind falls into. You might find yourself reaching into the future—you're sitting here and thinking, *This meditation stuff is really helpful, I wonder how I'll describe it to my wife, she'll think I'm crazy, she'll tell me I spent too much time living in California, it would be nice to take a vacation out there again soon*...And then remind yourself, there I was, off in fantasy, now I'm returning to focus on my breathing again.

You might find yourself wrestling with problems. You've followed two or three breaths, and then you're thinking, *What I'm going to do is call all his teachers. And then I'll say to them, you have to help him more, he doesn't know how to keep track of his homework. But that one teacher, the difficult one, she doesn't understand. Maybe I need to talk to the principal instead. That's it, that's what I'll do.* And then remind yourself again and return to focus on your breathing.

In other moments, you might spend time lost in the past. Rehashing the day, the week, or your life. *If only I hadn't said I was disappointed he lost his homework, I said I wouldn't give him a hard time anymore, he was so upset and now he isn't doing any of his homework at all, what I should have done was kept my mouth shut.* Notice those patterns as well, and then come back to the present.

Thoughts may reflect reality. We may choose to respond to them, and they may solve specific problems. But for these few minutes, notice the thoughts as "just thoughts," letting them pass through your mind likes clouds across a clear blue sky.

During the time you choose to sit, you're giving yourself time to step back, to not fix things. You're letting yourself settle down. Notice the problem-solving as thought as well, and let that go. You're sitting and nothing more.

It's amazing how easily minds wander off. It will happen, again and again. But both in the session and throughout your day, you can bring your attention back whenever you notice you've become lost. Break the endless cycle of mental and emotional chaos and instead return your attention to the world around you.

CHAPTER 9

Medical Options
for ADHD

*M*edications are not a magic pill, but they promote dramatic improvements in children with ADHD by addressing an intrinsic neurological
difference. These treatments for ADHD have been around for nearly seventy
years and are remarkably safe and effective. And regardless of what you may
have heard or feared, if you don't like their effects, stopping their use typically
allows side effects to resolve that day.

❧

The Foundation of ADHD Care

The concept of medication and children with ADHD has become a polar-
ized debate, and some people question whether ADHD medications are
appropriate in any situation. Yet the goal of medication in ADHD treatment is the same as with countless other medical conditions: to restore a
physiologic balance in the body. With ADHD, the imbalance is caused
by a deficiency in the frontal lobes of the brain, and there are no known
non-medical interventions that reverse this basic fact.

Refusing to even consider the biological cause of ADHD ignores the
research. Expecting someone with ADHD to be focused or less impulsive through purely behavioral means is like saying to someone with diabetes, "Make insulin already." It is not likely to resolve their situation.

At the same time, no one need advocate *for* medication any more
than people need to advocate *against*. When someone starts to have
problems with blood sugar control, doctors often try dietary changes

first. If this fails, or if someone's symptoms are already severe enough, doctors prescribe insulin. No well-trained doctor wants to give medications unnecessarily.

The same cautious approach works for ADHD. When there's room to try behavioral intervention alone, start there. Medication can be the last option for treating ADHD symptoms, as for many medical ailments. But from the point of view of a child hampered in life by an underactive part of their brain, there may be a rationale for early medical intervention as well.

Ideally, medications offer children with ADHD an ability to be their "best self" more often—calmer, less reactive, and more focused. It is inherently unfair to expect someone with a neurologically based disorder to overcome it through effort and will power alone. Medications, used properly, offer nothing more than an enhanced ability to monitor the same thoughts and impulses a child always has had.

Despite gains that often follow from behavioral and educational interventions, many professionals who treat ADHD consider medication the foundation of care. The defining symptoms of ADHD, such as hyperactivity, impulsiveness, distractibility, and poor focus, do not usually resolve without medication. When these impairments are severe or have persisted in spite of other attempts to tackle them, medications offer children an opportunity to thrive when they would otherwise struggle.

Still, any approach to ADHD care limited to one resource—medical, behavioral, or otherwise—misses an opportunity for more comprehensive growth. For families who choose medication, other problems often persist—challenges with relationships, learned habits that predate medication, and executive-function related difficulties with organization and long-term planning. Other conditions—such as reading disabilities or anxiety—frequently coexist with ADHD and require their own intensive interventions. To help the whole child, parents and children must adopt more than an "either this or that" attitude toward care.

A Child's Perspective

It's been amazing to watch. So many things have fallen into place. He's so much happier. He and my husband are playing together on the weekends like they never did. He's getting along with other kids better. He's

happy at school. Even piano has gotten better. He's so present and in the
moment. I feel like I gave him his childhood back.

cᴏ✖ᴏ

With successful medical intervention, a child with ADHD maintains self-regulation during the day. Whatever moments you have seen over time of their "best self"—joyful, relaxed in play and engaged at school—become possible on a consistent basis. They are the same person, but more in control and more at ease with the world.

Even when a child with untreated ADHD appears calm on the surface, the amount of energy needed to keep up with life can be exhausting. A student with passing grades and the ability to sit quietly in the classroom may suffer under the weight of the sheer effort spent compensating for their executive function difficulties. They may need to work five or ten times harder to accomplish as much as other classmates.

Living with ADHD is like fighting a continual battle with the brain. It takes grueling levels of exertion to overcome distractibility, forgetfulness, and keep track of all the details of life. In spite of the most genuine intentions, kids forget to take their homework to school. Or to take out the garbage. Or they impulsively push a child, or say something nasty when angry.

By starting ADHD medication, you are treating a specific condition and giving your children an opportunity to manage their own behavior. Medications, used properly, are not meant to ease the lives of parents, teachers, or anyone else, Their only place in treatment is to support the fundamental growth of children.

The Facts about ADHD Medication

While there are several types of ADHD medications, they all work by addressing the underlying differences in the frontal lobes. The most widely studied of this group, the stimulants, have that name because they preferentially "stimulate" an underactive area of the brain. Other medications do them same, acting to improve function in the frontal lobes through different biochemical mechanisms.

By causing the frontal lobes and related structures to be more responsive, we allow kids to more appropriately self-monitor. They maintain activities or interactions to their conclusion, instead of stopping mid-stride. Creativity, in many ways, is enhanced; instead of a child having many scattered ideas that never come to fruition, they define a single project with a beginning, middle, and end. Children have the same thoughts and impulses as ever, but modulate them and make more skillful choices.

Opponents of ADHD medications sometimes claim these treatments alter kids' personalities, but this is far from the truth. What ADHD medications really offer children is a skill they lack that most peers already have—the ability to self-regulate. This helps children direct their own behavior, stay on task in school and in play, and follow their plans through to the end. With a good medication fit, children often remark that they feel *more* like themselves—happier, at ease, and better able to control their own behavior.

To date, studies show no long-term detrimental effects from taking ADHD medication—but the benefits are profound. Underactive frontal lobes disrupt multiple paths of development throughout the brain and may limit any aspect of learning, from play skills to reading to tying a shoe. And then, as we reviewed in chapter four, unused neurons are trimmed away and learning opportunities lost. Medications, however, permit typical functioning for extended periods of time, and skills persist even after medications are no longer used. So while parents wonder about harmful effects of stimulants on the brain, more likely what appears is that by allowing better self-regulation, far-reaching areas of the brain develop to their potential.

What the Research Says

Studies of ADHD interventions are strikingly clear. One of the largest, referred to as the Multimodal Treatment of ADHD (MTA) study, randomly placed children with ADHD into three main groups: an intensive behavioral intervention group, a group that used only medication, and a group that used both behavior intervention and medication.[1]

It may sound intuitive that combined medication and behavior therapy would be the best outcome. Adding targeted counseling to medications should, on the surface, raise the intensity of intervention. Yet instead, the study showed a small benefit from behavior therapy for core ADHD symptoms (such as distractibility, hyperactivity and impulsivity), with a huge benefit from medication. There was little advantage to adding behavioral therapy to medication, as children who received either medication alone or the combined services did equally well.

Behavioral intervention in the MTA study had a clear role regarding broader ADHD care, helping with issues such as anxiety or poor self-esteem. Parents of children in the behavioral groups were happier—not a trivial finding, and one that offers guidance for parents and clinicians. In addition, the group receiving combined therapy required slightly lower stimulant doses.

A separate study using brain scans found "normalization" of functions within various brain regions affected by ADHD after one year on medication.[2] Children taking medication whose school performance was tracked over several years showed improved reading and math performance compared to children not taking medication. Other researchers compared two groups of pre-adolescents with ADHD, all of whom were off medication at the time.[3] Children who had taken medication at a younger age were functioning better than those who had never taken the medication; this finding suggests that children who take medication in their earlier years are less likely to need it when they get older.

While medication does not cure all the executive function deficits inherent in ADHD, it does appear to help these skills develop. A 2008 study comparing children who had taken ADHD preparations with those who had not found beneficial brain changes as a result of taking medication. The benefits included gains in executive function skills, attention, and handwriting. The children all were evaluated after being taken off medication; any benefits, therefore, were likely due to actual changes in the brain.[4]

Other research shows the incidence of oppositional behaviors decreases in children who begin medications at a young age, and that it is less likely that children taking medication will develop a full-blown diagnosis of oppositional defiant disorder.[5] Stimulant medications taken as a child may decrease the risk of ADHD-related anxiety or depression from developing later in life. Teens who take stimulant medications are at decreased risk for driving accidents and substance abuse. In all these different ways, new habits and abilities become hard-wired through ADHD treatment.[6]

Medication Myths

No one should ever take unneeded medications. And no medication exists without a potential for causing side effects. But the concept of medication has become unnecessarily terrifying to many parents. Beyond the fog of ADHD misinformation in the world, the basic facts are much more reassuring.

Stimulant-type ADHD medications have been around since the 1940s and tens of millions of people have taken them. It is unlikely there are major surprises waiting for discovery. And the only common side effects we know of resolve, usually the same day the medication is stopped.

ADHD medications do not accumulate in the body, so they pass through in a few hours. If they work, you must take them every day. When medications cause troublesome side effects, we discontinue them. Medication doesn't feel right? Call your doctor and make a change.

Medication should not alter personalities or sedate children. Kids still choose their own behaviors. The goal of medication is not to modify how children think or feel, or change who they are.

ADHD medications also are not addictive. In fact, the bigger risks are substance abuse and early alcohol use in people with *untreated* ADHD. Medical intervention for ADHD actually appears to *decrease* the risk of substance abuse over time.[7]

People sometimes state that they do not want to "medicate" their child. There is an implied message that as adults we impose our will, trying to reach out and alter a personality. But that is not the goal of quality care. When doctors prescribe medications for asthma, eczema, and ear infections, they *treat* those children. A better perspective question is, "What are the possible side effects of using medication, compared with the benefits of treating ADHD?"

Risks and Benefits

I think the medications are really working now. I can listen to my teacher, and I feel much happier. I'm even getting to do the extra assignment she gives us on Fridays.

⌒∞⌒

Deciding to use or not to use medication is not a trivial decision. The stakes feel huge. On an emotional level, someone prescribing a medication for what feels like a behavioral condition may chafe.

Horror stories float around the Internet, or make news headlines. Parents complain that they never find articles refuting the hyperbole and that shine a light on medication success stories. Medications pulled from the market make front page headlines and when found safe and returned to the shelves, the story is buried on page forty.

In reality, the side effects of having ADHD turn out to be more common than those induced by the medications. Untreated ADHD increases the likelihood of multiple developmental, academic, and social challenges. Young children with ADHD are at increased risk for falling behind academically. School dropout rates increase two- to threefold, as does the likelihood of job loss later in life.[8]

ADHD can disturb social development. As children mature, more prolonged verbal interactions become the norm, as does a degree of self-control and conversational focus. All are frequently disrupted by behaviors such as impulsivity or distractibility, as well as by impairments in executive function.[9] Children with ADHD often have significant trouble maintaining friendships, or have strained relationships with their parents.[10]

Children with ADHD are at two- to threefold risk for injuries, such as falls, bike accidents, or car crashes. As mentioned earlier, young children with ADHD seem more prone to emergency room visits due to random injuries. Without intervention, teens with ADHD are at much greater risk for impulsive behaviors such as early drinking, drug use, and promiscuity. And with ADHD, the cost of overall medical care more than doubles, perhaps because of ADHD-related difficulties with treatment compliance.[11]

But most of these risks may return to near baseline—the same as any other child or teenager—with a broad approach that includes family-based, educational, and medical care. When ADHD symptoms are under control, children are more available to learn from parents, teachers, and therapists. Behavioral interventions and parenting techniques that failed consistently in the past may become effective. Kids develop new skills and reach their potential in other aspects of life.

These facts are not meant to scare anyone into using the medications. The goal is balanced decision making, considering the implications of medication alongside what it means to be an individual going through life with ADHD. Having examined the effects ADHD has on your child, you still may decide not to use medications. That may be the most skillful path for your family, as long as you have looked at the situation with clarity and objectivity.

One common question parents have is whether medications become a crutch. They wonder if their child "needs to learn how to cope" with ADHD symptoms. But the opposite turns out to be true. By offering them the self-regulation to manage their own behavior, children learn and grow in ways they may not have otherwise. Even when kids stop medication, many of the skills they gained while on it still persist. Although further research is needed, using medications early in treatment may increase the chance they will not be needed later.

Choosing a Medication

After seventy years, stimulant medications like Ritalin remain the first line ADHD option. All the stimulants have the same potential benefits and side effects, with one class based on methylphenidate and one group based on (but not the same as) amphetamine. While any individual may sing the praise of one or the other brand, in reality they are interchangeable apart from length of effect.

Doctors often start kids with the longer-acting formulations, which last ten to twelve hours or more, but any individual may respond for much shorter lengths of time. Twice daily dosing or use of an additional short-acting medicine in the morning or afternoon is sometimes a great help to children. The goal is to find a medication that covers at a minimum breakfast to dinner.

COMMON ADHD MEDICATIONS

Stimulants:

Ritalin (methylphenidate)
Ritalin LA
Metadate CD/ER
Methylin
Daytrana
Dexidrine
Adderall
Adderall XR
Vyvanse
Focalin
Focalin XR

Second Line / Non-Stimulants:

Strattera (atomoxitine)
Tenex / guanfacine
Intuniv (guanfacine extended release)
Clonidine

Third Line:

Wellbutrin
Nortriptyline (and other anti-depressants)

Atomoxitine (Strattera) is often the next selection after the stimulants. Like stimulants, it works on pathways related to frontal lobe functioning, but while stimulants encourage the release of neurotransmitters in the brain, atomoxitine slows how quickly nerve cells reuse one. Atomoxitine is effective for ADHD control, but does not work as often as stimulants. However, it does not typically exacerbate issues with anxiety or tics, so it is sometimes the first medication prescribed for patients with ADHD and either of these comorbid conditions.

Atomoxitine takes four to six weeks to reach its peak effect, so decisions about effectiveness become more protracted. Once it works, however, it offers twenty-four-hour coverage. This can be a major benefit for teenagers and young adults who want to get their work done late at night. It also benefits children whose difficulty with self-regulation and planning makes an unremitting emotional mess of family time. Consistently painful mornings and nights are not a trivial part of child development, especially when they begin to define family relationships and self-concept.

Although the goal of treatment is to find a single medication that works, atomoxitine does not interact with the stimulants and is safe to use in combination. This may be useful because of added benefits when one or the other class of medication does not offer adequate coverage of ADHD on its own. Also, as a way of avoiding or minimizing side effects, atomoxitine may allow smaller stimulant doses to be effective.

Overall, atomoxitine tends to have fewer side effects than the stimulants, including less frequent trouble with appetite or sleep. It can cause symptoms such as stomach upset and headache. It may also potentially induce a list of emotional and mental health concerns similar to stimulants.

Guanfacine (Tenex), along with a related medication, clonidine, are blood pressure medications that benefit ADHD symptoms. Intuniv, a once-daily dosing of guanfacine, was released in 2009. These medications may have a particular benefit for patients susceptible to stimulant-induced irritability, and may help address sleep problems. They also can decrease tics and may be the first-choice medication for children with ADHD along with tics or Tourette's syndrome. Potential side effects include sedation, constipation, and, although rare, issues with blood pressure; side effects occur less frequently with Tenex and Intuniv than clonidine. At the doses used for

ADHD care, none of these three choices typically cause large changes in pressure.

Some antidepressants, such as Wellbutrin, may improve ADHD symptoms. They are most useful in patients who have symptoms of depression along with attention problems. Presently, they are used rarely for ADHD, in part because of an increased risk of side effects compared to other medicines.

Dealing with Side Effects

Without discounting the fact that adverse reactions are possible, the rate of side effects for ADHD medication is similar to many commonly used medications. Persistent issues are avoidable through the trial and error of finding the best selection for your child. There are several controversies, all of which will be reviewed shortly, but the overall success rate and safety has been consistently documented for decades.

The stimulants are not stored in the body. Their length of effect is several hours—from as little as three or four, to as many as twelve. They are not addictive, and they do not typically need weaning when stopped. The only reason someone should continue with a stimulant medication in spite of a significant side effect is as a rational choice—perhaps their overall life is greatly improved, in spite of a mild concern.

Sometimes when side effects are minimal, we decide to continue medications because the benefits are far greater. But if side effects are severe, all you need to do is contact the prescribing physician. With patient, systematic management, the vast majority of children will find a good fit among one of many available options.

⁂

We manage all the common side effects of stimulants through trying various formulations and fine-tuning dosages. The most commonly discussed issue with ADHD medications is appetite loss; it is also the hardest one to eliminate. However, their effects last only through the day, with a goal of coverage morning to early evening. Most children's bodies know their caloric needs and without thinking, the kids eat a little more at breakfast and dinner. Encourage healthy, calorie-dense snacks, especially once appetites kick back in after the medication leaves the system at night. While there can be some weight loss at the beginning of treatment, most children return to their normal growth patterns after several months.

As a side note, there is a high incidence of being overweight in untreated children with ADHD, most likely due to a combination of impulsivity and poor self-monitoring. With better self-regulation, eating habits improve. What looks like medication-related weight loss may actually be the child reaching a healthier equilibrium.

When stimulant medications last too long into the night, they can induce sleep difficulties. These problems may outlast any stimulant benefits seen during the day. Switching to shorter-acting medication resolves the issue most of the time. However, before stopping the medication because of sleep problems, consider your child's past patterns. A high number of children with ADHD have trouble with sleep in general, and upon reflection you may realize your child has never really slept well.[12] In fact, a small number of people with ADHD sleep better with the stimulants, with their mind and bodies more settled at night.

When starting medication some kids might experience mild physical discomfort like headaches or stomach upset. Small increases in heart rate or blood pressure may occur, though not typically a significant change for a child. While benefits do not vary over time, these mild side effects often improve on their own. Because of this, before deciding to discontinue treatment it may be best to give mild issues a short amount of time to diminish or disappear. Do not stop the medication without speaking to your child's doctor first, but when any side-effect becomes problematic, as always adjustments will be made.

The goal of medications is to help a child feel happier, less anxious, and more at ease in their life. In the process of trying ADHD medications, almost any behavior we hope to see improve can get worse, but only for as long as the medication is continued. If there is a clear emotional side effect even on day one, medications typically will be stopped or adjusted until a child feels better.

For the length of an individual dose, medications can make children anxious, jittery, irritable or quick to cry, separate from other tendencies they have. These emotional side effects traits can be hard to track. ADHD predisposes kids to be reactive, but the medications can themselves cause irritability or anxiety. And some kids do great on medications until the end of the day and then have a behavioral "rebound," a short stretch of time where symptoms worsen. This phenomena is avoidable for most by fine-tuning or switching their medicines.

A CONVERSATION FOR YOUR DOCTOR

As with any medication for any medical condition, the decision to take a drug should be based on a discussion with your doctor about its pros and cons. The information in this book is meant as an overview, and full details will be reviewed for you by a prescribing physician. If you choose to search for information on the Internet, only use reliable and unbiased sources.

Even the potential "rebound" can be confusing to define. Sometimes, improved behavior through the day becomes familiar, and what seems like an end-of-day escalation is actually a return to life without medication. However, when there is a clear "rebound," modifying the medication schedule should resolve the issue.

A good way to establish patterns is to keep notes in a calendar. ADHD-based reactivity or anxiety should be unchanged or improved by medication. Medication-induced side effects should be worse at the peak of the day's dosage. And rebound occurs at the end of the day.

If a child has a psychiatric condition in addition to ADHD, it can either improve or worsen with stimulant medications. Because these conditions often develop later in life, we do not always know which kids have a tendency for obsessive-compulsive disorder, anxiety, mania, psychosis, or any other mental health disorder. There also is a rare risk of other psychiatric side effects with these medications. But stimulants do not, as far as we know, cause long-term mental health problems. Stopping treatment should return children to wherever they were beforehand.

People often believe that a dulled personality is inevitable with ADHD treatment. Or that the goal is to tranquilize kids, to make them submissive. Might these side effects occur as modifications are made, for a day or several days? Absolutely. But if parents and providers are on the lookout, this is another unacceptable, and avoidable, side effect.

Several rare but severe side effects may be possible when using stimulant medications. Researchers have not yet reached a consensus about how often they occur, or if they happen at all. The three most discussed controversies are a possible slowing of growth, cardiac effects, and the worry that stimulants exacerbate tics.

Most studies do not find any long-term difference in height in children taking stimulants; for example, a 2010 study in the Journal of Pediatrics followed children ten years into early adulthood and found no differences.[13] Some researchers suggest there is an initial slowing when starting stimulants in some children, but that catch-up growth occurs later. Practically, monitoring the growth curve (the percentiles pediatricians watch for in any child) reassures most families that growth remains on track.[14]

Stimulants do not damage healthy hearts, as far as research has shown to date. Comprehensive studies have shown no increase in the risk for cardiac-related events (such as heart attacks) in children taking stimulants.[15] Only controversial reports have described a slight statistical risk for children taking stimulants, with methods and data interpretations that have been debated.

Children with heart disease may be monitored more closely while taking stimulants. Because of this, children who have fainted or experienced any symptoms possibly related to heart disease are usually screened before starting medication, as are children with a family history of early-onset heart disease, or those with relatives who had heart troubles early in life.[16]

Lastly, people debate whether stimulants may or may not exacerbate tics, such as uncontrollable vocalizations or muscle twitches. Recent studies have shown no relationship between use of stimulants and frequency of tics, and their frequency may in fact *decrease* in some patients while taking stimulants. In addition, children with ADHD are at higher risk for tic disorders in general; new onset tics may occur coincidently after beginning stimulants, when they would have started on their own.

However, it does remain possible that stimulant use exacerbates tics for some children.[17] One difference from other side effects is that the natural course for tics is to come and go over days or weeks once they begin. Because of that, unlike the rest of the side effects on the list, tics can last for a time after discontinuing the medication. However, if problems occur, they typically resolve when medication use stops.

Apart from poor appetite, if you have ever heard of someone with ADHD living indefinitely with medication side effects, that person either falls in the small group of children who do not tolerate the medications, or who need an adjustment. As mentioned, sometimes the benefits of medication are so great that even with minor side effects, people choose to continue them. But if you observe persistent troubles in your child, talk with your physician as there is quite likely another, better-tolerated option that could help.

Managing Medication

I told my child, of course you're smart. You are smarter than most kids, and you are amazingly creative and have all these thoughts going on that are exciting and artistic and fun. Your mind is busy. The medication doesn't make you smart. It's more like a traffic cop. It says to you, hold on a second, first focus over here, get this done . . . and now run off and play.

⚬❧⚬

The art of prescribing medication is about close follow-up and frequent fine-tuning. Dosing of ADHD medications does not depend on weight or choosing a specific medication to start. Small children respond to large doses, big people respond to small doses. Some people respond better to one medication, some to others. Medication doses can move up and down. Switching between the various stimulant medications may also continue until symptoms are well controlled. There is no better answer for these trials than patience, and arriving at a good place is a matter of constant adjusting. And then kids change, and you need to correct again.

The effects of most ADHD medications are immediate. For stimulants, day one benefits will be the same as day one hundred. Of course, other things affect kids' behavior day to day, so we cannot attribute every high or low to the medication. As well, benefits and side effects may be subtle at first—a slight drop in distractibility, or a vague, one-time headache. But once a response is clear, usually over a few days, another change can be made.

Earlier in this chapter we reviewed the MTA study, which showed the benefits of medication compared to behavioral intervention. The study contained a fourth group of children diagnosed with ADHD and then returned to the community for treatment. Instead of remaining in one of the main study groups, their general pediatricians made whatever choices they felt best for care.

This community treatment group did not do as well as the children who received medication through the MTA study. But why? Within the MTA, the protocol was for constant modification of the medications until the children either reached full control of ADHD symptoms or encountered side effects. When side effects started, the dose was scaled back or the medication changed.

In the community, physicians and parents instead tended to leave doses at the same level as whenever they first noticed a benefit. After years of rampant hyperactivity or poor focus, a little improvement began on a small dose. Everyone involved was likely thrilled. But probably, ADHD symptoms persisted and hindered learning or socialization. Wise medication use involves knowing when to try a little more, with a willingness to step back and make a change again.

❦

When medications function well, people choose to take them every day. While people often view ADHD as only a school problem, it affects a child's relationship with peers and with adults who out of necessity may give near constant feedback when correcting and redirecting behavior. It affects self-esteem and ego development, as children wrestle with their own inability to keep track of their responsibilities and daily lives.

Benefits extend far beyond school hours as multiple aspects of life fall into place, along with an enhanced ability to learn from parents, teachers, therapists, friends, and their own experience. Children become calmer and more at ease, social situations become more fluid and easier. Work gets done more smoothly and kids misplace or forget things less often. Kids feel less reactive, and are less likely to say or do something impulsively.

For all of these reasons, ADHD medications most often are prescribed daily, including weekends. There is no physical need for a weekend break unless there is a persistent side effect, such as weight loss. In fact, if someone does not want to take their medication Saturday and Sunday, this desire to skip days may be an indication that their medications are not yet right.

Seven days a week is not a hard and fast rule for stimulants, however, as it is medically safe to start and stop them. It may be helpful to take some notes, comparing a few days at home on and off the medication. If they are old enough to notice, ask children how they feel about the decision. Many are quite clear at a relatively young age if they prefer taking it. Note the quality of interactions your child has with you, with siblings, and with friends. If there is truly no difference between on and off, discuss with your physician what to do next.

Guidelines for Monitoring and Adjusting Medications

Set clear treatment goals. As you would probably guess, if you expect every social, academic, or oppositional behavior to fall into place right away, you may be disappointed. ADHD medications primarily improve symptoms such as poor focus, distractibility, activity level, and impulsivity, and often emotional reactivity as well; they do not affect as directly the broader list of executive function difficulties reviewed in chapter three. Setting clear target goals with your physician along these lines will help with long-term management. The ADHD rating scales mentioned on page 30 provide good guidelines for monitoring; others also have value and may be preferred by various clinicians.

Adjust medications frequently. Stimulant medications have their full effect the day they start. Some mild side effects may get better, but generally what you see is what you get and after a week or less adjustments can be made. Occasionally, a child begins medication and changes in an instant, from that exact prescription; one of the most gratifying experiences providers have is when families return glowing after a week or two. The fighting is gone, parents and children are happy, and that's that. But this is the exception, and while medications significantly improve ADHD symptoms, they commonly require time and fine-tuning. Other medications, like Strattera, need time to reach their peak impact, with reassessment after several weeks.

Monitor medication timing. There is a lifestyle to living with ADHD medications, especially the stimulants. They peak in their effectiveness between thirty and ninety minutes after being taken. Their effects generally wane anywhere from four to twelve hours later.

When laying out a daily schedule, keep track of these patterns. Homework is best done while the medication is working. Adjustments in medications can increase coverage later in the afternoon or early evening, or allow for a faster onset in the morning. As frustrating as it may be for a child or a parent, a schedule that consistently forces homework or other challenging activities into unmedicated nighttime hours may be destined to fail.

Get information from teachers, in addition to your own input. The timing of medications varies greatly from product to product, and from child to child. What lasts for twelve hours for one child might last another seven. Parents do not always observe the height of the medication, which five days a week occurs during school hours. Benefits and side effects may be gone by the end of the day. Both teacher information and direct observation by parents guide care.

If symptoms do not change over time, reevaluate. ADHD symptoms improve with medication in 80 percent of children, or more. That still means approximately one in five will not benefit from medication, so a disappointing response from a medication trial does not necessarily mean more is going on than ADHD. However, two-thirds of people with ADHD have a related condition. When treatment stalls a poor response to medication is possible, but a reevaluation is needed to look for undetected behavioral or academic problems. And as there is no concrete ADHD test, you may want to consider the possibility that the diagnosis itself was not correct.

Periodically stop medications and reassess their benefits. Between symptoms returning at night as stimulant effectiveness wanes and parents forgetting or skipping doses on occasion, children experience time off medications and ADHD symptoms often returns to the forefront. But, as noted earlier, children may outgrow ADHD over several years. Where medications were a cornerstone of their development at age eight, by fifteen, symptoms may have improved to a point they no longer impair daily life.

If you are unclear whether your child still has ADHD at any given point, ask your physician about a trial period off medications. Typically this is done over the summer, outside of school. If it makes sense after those weeks, the upcoming school year can be started without medications, with close follow-up through the beginning of the year.

Alternative and Complementary Options

You may hear about a neighbor or friend of a friend or celebrity who had an experience, either good or bad, using an alternative treatment. Someone claims an herbal supplement cured their child, or that some other intervention caused their hair to turn purple. These emotionally charged vignettes often influence judgments.

On a practical level, some complementary interventions have been studied extensively and have evolved over decades. Some have budding research or solid theory behind them, while some already have research showing they do not work. Some make little sense theoretically once you understand the science of ADHD. And in the broadest sense, the most effective non-medical care is the parent or teacher-based interventions reviewed in chapters seven and eight.

Some commonly discussed complementary interventions include:

Dietary Changes

Controlled studies of sugar intake use an odd placebo. The sugar pill, which in medicine normally is given to the group not being treated, becomes the intervention. When adults do not know which children in a group have ingested sugar and which have not, they cannot tell the difference between behaviors. In spite of all the anecdotal stories, sugar does not seem to influence behavior.[18]

Studies of brightly colored food additives suggest they increase hyperactivity in some children, although this effect is not large enough to cause ADHD.[19] Without a major upheaval in life, you can observe your child. If after eating or drinking artificial food dyes her behavior changes, restrict these items. Or, since these products have limited nutritional value to start, cut them out anyway.

Correcting true nutritional deficiencies, such as low levels of iron and possibly zinc, may improve attention. This does not mean supplements improve attention in otherwise healthy children. Likewise, some studies show taking fish oil or omega-3 fatty acids benefits attention, and other studies found it makes no difference at all. If there is benefit to omega-3 fatty acids it likely hinges on making sure kids get at least the adequate minimum, ideally through food and never through megadoses.

Restriction diets, such as the gluten-free diet, have been a recent trend in alternative care. There is no evidence they affect ADHD symptoms.

Attention Training

Since motivated adults can build attention skills through specific mental exercises, people often wonder how to use the same techniques for children. Without erasing the underlying ADHD, several studies have shown that kids can benefits from meditation instruction or related mindfulness techniques for ADHD symptoms and executive function. Working individually or in groups, programs that teach meditation or yoga to young children appear to improve attention, emotional regulation, executive function, and related skills. As mentioned earlier, completed studies have revealed benefits down through elementary school for mindfulness training, and in younger children with play-based interventions.[20]

Exactly when and how to begin this type of training is open for debate. But research points in the same direction. As a whole, children benefit from an early emphasis on social emotional abilities.

On a basic level, you start by modeling mindfulness in daily life yourself. Demonstrate what you want your children to learn about how to live their lives. Focus your lifestyle on free play and other unstructured activities that support the development of self-regulation and problem-solving abilities.

Beginning there, you can teach anything you have read about in this book to your kids, modifying for age and interest. Pausing before acting. Taking a few breaths when angry, or taking time to yourself. Eating with intention. Noticing what is going on in their environment. Describing and accepting emotional states as they arise. Living with compassion and respect for others. Creating for yourself the language, brevity, and cultural adaptations that fit your child. Susan Kaiser-Greenland's book *The Mindful Child* describes many accessible, entertaining ways to introduce mindfulness to children.

Computer Training and Neurofeedback

Computer training and neurofeedback strive to take advantage of neuroplasticity and attention training in a similar fashion. Various products are available that claim improvement in attention and executive function through use of specially designed computer activities. Neurofeedback allows individuals to observe their own physiological functioning, such as through use of an electroencephalogram (EEG), and then attempts to show them how to modify these central nervous system measures. Some studies suggest both may be useful for training skills such as attention and working memory.[21] No studies suggest they can replace medication or other interventions.

Presently, the exact details for these programs—how they should be implemented and with whom—remains ill-defined, and they can be expensive. But as long as they avoid creating unrealistic expectations for families and do not replace other forms of care, they do not appear harmful.

Exercise

Several small studies suggest a benefit from exercise. Afternoon behavior in school tends to be better in children with a regularly scheduled recess.[22] Another study even showed benefit for outdoor versus indoor activity, as the same exercise routine improved ADHD symptoms more when done in a park.[23] If your child appears to benefit from exercise, schedule it as part of the day throughout the year, remembering that 'exercise' for a child means anything from a structured class to free time on the playground or in the back yard.

Auditory and Vision Training

Auditory processing issues in ADHD, which are discussed in chapter 3, relate to poor executive function and attention abilities, until proven otherwise. Interventions based on the auditory system therefore do not improve ADHD. Similarly, the American Academy of Pediatrics recently released a policy statement and research summary regarding vision training. Visual interventions do not resolve ADHD, learning disabilities, or other behavioral problems.

Guidelines for Decision Making with Complementary Medicine

1. **First do no harm**. Some alternative interventions can be dangerous for children. Alternative medicine is regulated differently from prescription medicines and often not regulated at all, so you may not have a clear view of product ingredients or dose sizes. Biochemically active substances like St. John's Wort (which is used to treat depression in some countries) show up in everything from ADHD treatment to herbal teas. Mega-doses of nutritional supplements can cause illness. Something labeled "natural" or sold over the counter will not be appropriate or safe for all children.

2. **Evaluate the effect on the family.** If something safe and affordable works for you or your child, making you feel better or enhancing a particular skill set, acknowledge that. However, some interventions are brutally expensive with little evidence saying they work. Others, like intense dietary intervention, can be incredibly stressful and disruptive. Restricting a diet even further on a child with already limited tastes can be an emotional and nutritional mess. The benefits of many interventions are uncertain at best in spite of the logistical, financial, or emotional stresses they provoke.

3. **Understand the theory.** People often try to sell interventions that do not make sense on a theoretical level, and do not have evidence to back them up. ADHD is a condition caused by underactivity of a particular part of the brain. Something new could simply be ahead of the research, but when the theory is questionable you are at risk for buying snake oil. While we cannot explain the benefits of every technique, ask questions and think critically.

4. **Assess the benefits carefully.** Recognize that many things can help a child improve their behavior or attention. If your child starts a new school program that includes academic supports and

counseling, and then you try an ADHD medication, and you simultaneously try an alternative intervention, their symptoms may improve. But which piece of the plan helped most, and which not at all?

Medical Intervention and Mindfulness

Nothing is done *to* children when prescribing medication. A child with ADHD has behavioral problems rooted in biochemistry, so you offer them better self-regulation, and an opportunity to thrive. In making a medication decision—for or against—the most important step a parent can take is toward balanced objectivity.

Check your sources. Some authors and websites make wild claims, but the experiences of any individual or family do not generalize. When a neighbor's child responds in some extreme fashion it does not mean anyone else ever will. They might have another condition entirely, or have followed up poorly with their doctor, or have reacted with a one-in-a-million side effect.

A teacher may report that she's seen kids turn their lives around with medications, or alternatively that medication turns them into zombies. Again, that's her small sliver of the picture. Our own experience only goes so far; if my life were changed by winning the lottery, would you depend on changing yours the same way?

It is easy to get swept up in anxiety, carried away by stories you have heard. Your belief systems around behavior, effort, and ADHD have been developing your whole life. Notice when you become fixed in your thinking, and pause. Try to see the decision without reactivity, and with insight.

If you feel you lack information find an expert to ask, or two. Perhaps some side effect concerns you; how often does it occur, and how at risk is your child? Perhaps you are unclear about the benefits, or the effect, of medication on the body. Ask questions until you have a clear picture of the pluses and minuses.

All you can ever do, with any choice, is make the best decision you can, right now. What is going on for your child? Is the diagnosis valid? Why are they still struggling in spite of everything else you have tried? What problems is ADHD causing, and what problems can the medications cause?

In any moment, step out of autopilot and act with clear intention. Respond with whatever wisdom you can muster. Once you have decided, look back at the outcome and try not to judge yourself for it. You have made the best choice you could, by definition. And then with mindfulness and objectivity, reflect. Did it work out like you expected? Sometimes it will, and sometimes it will not. Giving yourself a break, and without self-recrimination, try again. Right now, today, what makes sense to do next?

CHAPTER 10

Supporting the Whole Family

Y ou've taken a step in a new direction, toward broader ADHD care, inner resilience, and family peace. Your child is unlikely to have been the one to come to you and say, "I need more routines. Please Dad, use more consistency when you set limits for me." Or, "Mom, maybe a structured reward system would help me get it together." You were the one who took the first steps down a new road. And this is good news—you decided when the time for change had arrived.

Accepting the reality of ADHD as a chronic medical condition, you have started to make clear-sighted decisions not driven by reactivity or fearfulness. In a world of frequently skewed information, choices that take care of yourself and your family are free of bias and misinformation. The first step toward reclaiming family life, therefore, was to objectively decide: Is this ADHD? If you already knew that your child had ADHD, or in reading this book you have decided that they do, there may have been basic assumptions to reconsider. Failing to do homework or to behave well because you *cannot* is different than because you *will* not.

The beginning decision is often about medication management. You may try other interventions first, but recognize at the same time that the research on medication is clear. When ADHD is correctly diagnosed and impairing some aspect of life, care most often requires addressing the biological differences underlying the behavioral symptoms. Used judiciously, ADHD medications uniquely control symptoms such as inattention, distractibility, impulsivity, and related emotional reactivity.

You may still be hearing the same stories about medications. They change personalities, stunt growth, or cause heart problems. Of course, the rumors trigger anxiety, but now you know the reality behind them. Pause and reflect, take a breath, and continue to search for the truth, to the best of your abilities. Stepping out of fear, what is the most practical decision you can make for your child, and your family?

Medication alone rarely addresses the full range of issues caused by this complex neurobiological condition. Most people with ADHD have executive function problems, and most have other educational or developmental conditions along with their ADHD. Executive function problems impact home life, school performance, and work, and cause children to fall behind developmentally. ADHD affects children's views of themselves and their relationships with others, areas of life requiring more than medical intervention to change.

Various parenting techniques, from refining your use of praise and reward to maintaining long-term consistency in your limit-setting, play an invaluable role at home. Responsive behavioral management, at times augmented with therapy and counseling, also affects child development and family life. Countless hard-to-quantify patterns may have persisted because they are habit, such as arguing, or defensiveness, or motivational issues. Co-existing problems like low self-esteem or anxiety may continue. But you can now meet your children right where they are in their development, and set up a plan to build skills gradually, over time.

School is a huge part of your child's life, and buttressed with knowledge about ADHD and executive function in the classroom, you can help educators see your child with the same objectivity and basic ADHD knowledge you have cultivated for yourself. If teachers consistently raise concerns about your child's behavior in class, you now can address them together. Seek out evaluation, push for appropriate supports, and make certain someone instructs your child in organizational skills.

In starting to explore mindfulness, you perhaps slowed down and paid attention to everything in more detail, or became a little more familiar with some of your habits, maybe finding some you like, and maybe some you dislike. Having done nothing else, you steered your whole family toward greater resilience and well-being.

You now have the knowledge and the tools you need to take control of ADHD. You understand the cause, and that the effects reach far beyond either "attention deficit" or "hyperactivity." You have all the information at hand to make tough choices about parenting, behavioral change, schooling, and medication. And through mindfulness, you have the methods to keep yourself mentally fit, flexible, and balanced, riding the waves without being pulled under.

Your ADHD Management Checklist

All of a sudden, I got it. Years of frustration about not being listened to evaporated. He had never heard. Once I realized what it really meant to have ADHD, our lives changed. He listens most of the time if I get his attention first. I don't ask as much at once. I've tried to show him what he can do for himself. I fall off the wagon once in a while, but everything is so much calmer.

⸎

Being the parent of a child with ADHD is very, very hard. Just because you now are able to approach your job with new knowledge and new skills doesn't mean you've done anything wrong in the past. Just because you're learning to manage your stress and challenges differently doesn't mean you've caused any of your difficulties before.

Parents of children with ADHD are uniquely challenged. Typical parenting styles and routines may not be effective. Expectations about being a parent, or what family life should be, have been thrown into turmoil. Life may feel out of control as you struggle to advocate for your children. Mindfulness returns a sense of strength and clarity in defining a new path, and adds more specific benefits for the entire family.

For children, life skills begin with stable homes, clear limit-setting, and an emphasis on free play and creativity, areas that may fall by the wayside in the face of ADHD, unless parents pay attention along the way. There also is the link between ADHD and attention training. An increasing body of evidence suggests that children benefit from activities that develop attention capacities, cognitive flexibility, and emotional resilience. While research with children around direct training is still in its infancy, it one day may widely augment traditional Western education and health care.

With the knowledge you culled from this book, you may already find yourself on more solid ground. What follows is a "top ten list" of reminders for managing family life, and ADHD. I hope you can use this list as an anchor, returning for reassurance and guidance whenever you sense ADHD is pulling you to sea.

1. **Maintain an understanding of ADHD biology and executive function.** Find clear, evidence-based sources of information and stick to them. Encourage other adults in your child's life to do the same.

2. **Emphasize strengths and successes.** For your own well-being and that of your children, even in the midst of challenging times pay attention to moments in which they thrive, seeking to create a world where they experience positive feedback far more than negative.

3. **Examine where your child struggles.** While not every challenge that crops up will prove to be rooted in ADHD, executive function impacts many aspects of life. If you feel yourself becoming angry because of behavior that seems willful or poorly motivated, step back for a moment, pause, and reflect. Reassess over time, allowing for the possibility of growth and addressing new issues when they develop.

4. **Objectively decide about medication.** What are the actual risks and potential benefits for your child? For children using medications, periodically pause and confirm with your physician that the medications are still needed and that dosages remain appropriate.

5. **Continue to polish your ADHD parenting skills.** Emphasize praise and reward balanced by consistent limits and routines, even when progress seems slow. Be aware of patterns in behavior. Manage concerns as they arise, noting what might be ADHD driven, and implement appropriate plans and immediate consequences as needed.

6. **Observe your parenting style with objectivity, and without self-judgment.** What skills might you further develop around consistency, limit setting, routines, behavioral management, or anything else?

7. **Collaborate with your child's school.** Listen to what teachers and other school staff have to say about your child. They are educational experts and can guide you and your children toward success. At the same time, having cultivated your own awareness of ADHD, strongly advocate for a program that takes your child's actual abilities into account and allows them to excel.

8. **Never expect to be the expert**. When plans are not effective, consider working with a trained professional, such as a physician, psychologist, or social worker. Head off emotional or behavioral concerns early. It's better to realize an intervention is no longer needed than to wait out a problem, only to see it solidify and grow.

9. **Take care of yourself.** Protect time that allows you to stay balanced, strong, and capable of making compassionate, wise decisions for your family. When you begin to feel overwhelmed, step back and make certain you've been doing what you need for yourself.

10. **Be mindful whenever and as often as you can.** The mindfulness exercises outlined throughout *The Family ADHD Solution* support you in taking a first step toward change. You may have experimented with them while you read, or you may have breezed through. Training in mindfulness requires dedication and time, so commit to taking care of yourself with a break, practicing meditation once or twice a day. Each and every time will not be peaceful and life-changing, but with persistence you'll focus your attention with more *intention*, and changes will follow.

❦

You can do nothing more or less as a parent than strive to change what you can, and to accept the rest. You guide children while also allowing them to find their own way through the world. You pause to enjoy the incremental improvements encountered along the way, without always pushing for more, refining skills while at the same time not expecting too much of your child, or yourself.

Moving forward, you have all the resources needed to lead your child and your family toward a less stressful, more successful future. Through insight into the inner workings of ADHD and the outer manifestations of this common condition, you will continue to make wise choices that benefit your children. May whatever tools you have found most useful in *The Family ADHD Solution* help you toward a life of happiness, health, and ease.

Suggested Resources

Barkley, Russell A. *Taking Charge of ADHD: The Complete, Authoritative Guide for Parents (Revised Edition).* New York and London: The Guilford Press, 2000.

———— and Christine M. Benton. *Your Defiant Child: Eight Steps to Better Behavior.* New York and London: The Guildford Press, 1998.

Begley, Sharon. *Train Your Mind, Change Your Brain: How a New Science Reveals Our Extraordinary Potential to Transform Ourselves.* New York: Ballantine Books, 2008.

Greene, Ross W. *The Explosive Child: A New Approach for Understanding and Parenting Easily Frustrated, Chronically Inflexible Children.* New York: Harper, 2010.

Greenland, Susan K. *The Mindful Child: How to Help Your Kid Manage Stress and Become Happier, Kinder, and More Compassionate.* New York: Free Press, 2010.

Kabat-Zinn, Jon. *Full Catastrophe Living: Using the Wisdom of Your Body and Mind to Face Stress, Pain, and Illness.* New York: Delta Trade Paperback, 2005.

————. *Guided Mindfulness Meditation CDs Series 1, 2 and 3.* Sounds True, Inc., 2005.

Phelan, Thomas W. *1–2–3 Magic: Effective Discipline for Children 2–12,* 3rd edition. Glen Ellyn, IL: ParentMagic, Inc., 2003.

Reiff, Michael I. and Sherill Tippins. *ADHD: A Complete and Authoritative Guide.* American Academy of Pediatrics, 2004.

Saltzman, Amy. *Still Quiet Place, Mindfulness for Young Children (2004)* and *Mindfulness for Teens (2010),* CDs of guided mindfulness exercises.

Salzberg, Sharon and Joseph Goldstein. *Insight Meditation: A Step-by-Step Course on How to Meditate.* Louisville, CO: Sounds True, Inc., 2006.

Siegel, Daniel J. *The Mindful Brain: Reflection and Attunement in the Cultivation of Well-Being.* New York and London: W. W. Norton and Company, 2007.

Weissbluth, Marc. *Happy Sleep Habits, Happy Child*. New York: Ballantine Books, 2005.

Zeigler Dendy, Chris A. *CHADD Educator's Manual on Attention Deficit/ Hyperactivity Disorder (AD/HD): An In-depth Look from an Educational Perspective*. CHADD (Children and Adults with Attention Deficit- Hyperactivity Disorder), 2006.

Notes

Chapter 1: ADHD, Parenting, and the Brain

1. Patricia N. Pastor and Cynthia A. Reuben, "Diagnosed Attention Deficit Hyperactivity Disorder and Learning Disability: United States, 2004–2006," National Center for Health Statistics, *Vital Health Statistics* 10(237).

2. Russell A. Barkley, *Attention-Deficit Hyperactivity Disorder: A Handbook for Diagnosis and Treatment*, 3rd ed. (New York: The Guilford Press, 2006), 98–108.

3. Guilherme Polanczyk, Maurício Silva de Lima, Bernardo Lessa Horta, Joseph Biederman, and Luis Augusto Rohde, "The Worldwide Prevalence of ADHD: A Systematic Review and Metaregression Analysis," *American Journal of Psychiatry* 164(6): 942–948.

4. For a review of twin studies, see Barkley, *Attention Deficit Hyperactivity Disorder*, 227–228.

5. Tanya E. Froehlich, Bruce P. Lanphear, Peggy Auinger, Richard Hornung, Jeffery N. Epstein, Joe Braun, and Robert S. Kahn, "Association of Tobacco and Lead Exposures with Attention-Deficit/Hyperactivity Disorder," *Pediatrics* 124(6): e1054-e1063. See also J. Gordon Millichap, "Etiologic Classification of Attention-Deficit/Hyperactivity Disorder," *Pediatrics* 121(2): e358-e365.

6. Nigel M. Williams, et al, "Rare Chromosomal Deletions and Duplications in Attention-Deficit Hyperactivity Disorder: A Genome-Wide Analysis," *The Lancet*, September 30, 2010.

7. Steven G. Dickstein, Katie F. Bannon, Xavier F. Castellanos, and Michael P. Milham, "The Neural Correlates of Attention-Deficit Hyperactivity Disorder: An ALE Meta-analysis," *Journal of Child Psychology and Psychiatry, and Allied Disciplines* 47(10): 1051–1062.

8. Russell A. Barkley, et al., "International Consensus Statement on ADHD," *Clinical Child and Family Psychology Review* 5(2): 89–111.

See also Steven G. Dickstein, Katie F. Bannon, Xavier F. Castellanos, and Michael P. Milham, "The Neural Correlates of Attention-Deficit Hyperactivity Disorder: An ALE meta-analysis," *Journal of Child Psychology and Psychiatry, and Allied Disciplines* 47(10): 1051–1062. See also Chandan J. Vaidya and Melanie Stollstorff, "Cognitive Neuroscience of Attention Deficit Hyperactivity Disorder: Current Status and Working Hypotheses," *Developmental Disabilities Research Reviews* 14(4): 261–267.

9. Russell A. Barkley, *ADHD and the Nature of Self-Control* (New York: The Guilford Press, 1997).

10. Mona M. Shattell, Robin Bartlett, and Tracie Rowe, "'I Have Always Felt Different': The Experience of Attention-Deficit/Hyperactivity Disorder in Childhood," *Journal of Pediatric Nursing* 23(1): 49–57.

11. Todd B. Kashdan, Rolf G. Jacob, William E. Pelham, Alan R. Lang, Betsy Hoza, Jonathan D. Blumenthal, and Elizabeth M. Gnagy, "Depression and Anxiety in Parents of Children with ADHD and Varying Levels of Oppositional Defiant Behaviors: Modeling Relationships with Family Functioning," *Journal of Clinical Child and Adolescent Psychology* 33(1): 169–181.

12. William B. Brinkman, Susan N. Sherman, April R. Zmitrovich, Marty O. Visscher, Lori E. Crosby, Kieran J. Phelan, and Edward F. Donovan, "Parental Angst Making and Revisiting Decisions about Treatment of Attention-Deficit/Hyperactivity Disorder," *Pediatrics* 124(2): 580–589.

13. Brian T. Wymbs, William E. Pelham, Jr., Brooke S. Molina, Elizabeth M. Gnagy, Tracey K. Wilson, and Joel B. Greenhouse, "Rate and Predictors of Divorce Among Parents of Youths with ADHD," *Journal of Consulting and Clinical Psychology* 76(5): 735–744.

Chapter 2: The Path to Diagnosis

1. Mark J. Sciutto and Miriam Eisenberg, "Evaluating the Evidence for and against the Overdiagnosis of ADHD," *Journal of Attention Disorders* 11(2): 106–113.

2. Elizabeth R. Sowell, et al, "In Vivo evidence for post-adolescent brain maturation in frontal and striatal regions," *Nature Neuroscience*, 2(20): 859–861; Nitin Gogtay, et al, "Dynamic mapping of human cortical development during childhood through early adulthood," *Proceedings of the National Academy of Sciences*, 101 (21): 8174–8179.

3. Helen Link Egger, Douglas Kondo, and Adrian Angold, "The Epidemiology and Diagnostic Issues in Preschool Attention-Deficit/ Hyperactivity Disorder: A Review," *Infants and Young Children* 19(2): 109–122.

4. Heather T. Keenan, Gillian C. Hall, and Stephen W. Marshall, "Early Head Injury and Attention Deficit Hyperactivity Disorder: Retrospective Cohort Study," *The British Medical Journal* 337(7680): a1984.

5. Steven M. Alessandri, "Attention, Play, and Social Behavior in ADHD Preschoolers," *Journal of Abnormal Child Psychology* 20(3): 289–302.

6. Adele Diamond, "Attention-deficit disorder (attention deficit/hyper-activity disorder without hyperactivity): A neurobiologically and behaviorally distinct disorder from attention deficit/hyperactivity disorder with hyperactivity," *Development and Psychopathology*, 17 (2005), 807–825.

7. Brendan F. Andrade, Darlene A. Brodeur, Daniel A. Waschbusch, Sherry H. Stewart, and Robin McGee, "Selective and Sustained Attention as Predictors of Social Problems in Children with Typical and Disordered Attention Abilities," *Journal of Attention Disorders* 12(4): 341–352.

8. For discussion of MRI and EEG diagnostic studies, see Russell A. Barkley, *Attention-Deficit Hyperactivity Disorder: A Handbook for Diagnosis and Treatment, 3rd ed.* (New York: The Guildford Press, 2006), 362.

9. Michael J. Kofler, Mark D. Rapport, Jennifer Bolden and Thomas A. Altro, "Working Memory as a Core Deficit in ADHD: Preliminary Findings and Implications," *The ADHD Report* 16(2008): 8–14.

10. Russell A. Barkley, *Attention-Deficit Hyperactivity Disorder: A Handbook for Diagnosis and Treatment*, 3rd ed. (New York: The Guildford Press, 2006), 377.

11. Ibid., 184.

12. Josephine Elia, Paul Ambrosini, and Wade Berrettini, "ADHD Characteristics: I. Concurrent Co-Morbidity Patterns in Children and Adolescents," *Child and Adolescent Psychiatry and Mental Health* 2(1): 15.

13. Susan D. Mayes, Susan L. Calhoun, and Erin W. Crowell, "Learning Disabilities and ADHD: Overlapping Spectrum Disorders," *Journal of Learning Disabilities* 33, no. 5 (September–October 2000): 417–24.

14. David R. Moore, et al., "Nature of Auditory Processing Disorder in Children," *Pediatrics* 2010:126, July 26, 2010, http://www.pediatrics.org/cgi/content/full/126/2/e382.

Chapter 3: ADHD Beneath the Surface

1. Although there are other ways of classifying the brain's various executive functions, I have adapted a formulation similar to the one found in Thomas E. Brown, "Executive: Describing Six Aspects of a Complex Syndrome," *Attention Magazine*, February 2008, 12–17.

2. Nora D. Volkow, Gene-Jack Wang, Scott H. Kollins, Tim L. Wigal, Jeffrey H. Newcorn, Frank Telang, Joanna S. Fowler, Wei Zhu, Jean Logan, Yeming Ma, Kith Pradhan, Christopher Wong, and James M. Swanson, "Evaluating Dopamine Reward Pathway in ADHD," *Journal of the American Medical Association* 2009; 302 (10): 1084–1091.

3. Julie Sarno Owens, Matthew E. Goldfine, Nicole M. Evangelista, Betsy Hoza and Nina M. Kaiser, "A Critical Review of Self-perceptions and the Positive Illusory Bias in Children with ADHD," *Clinical Child and Family Psychology Review* 10, no. 4 (2007): 335–351.

Chapter 4: Attention Training and the Brain

1. Gregg H. Recanzone, Christoph E. Schreiner, and Michael M. Merzenich, "Plasticity in the Frequency Representation of Primary Auditory Cortex Following Discrimination Training in Adult Owl Monkeys," *The Journal of Neuroscience* 13(1): 87–103.

2. Guinevere F. Eden, Karen M. Jones, Katherine Cappell, Lynn Gareau, Frank B. Wood, Thomas A Zeffiro, Nicole A. E. Dietz, John A. Agnew, and D. Lynn Flowers, "Neural Changes Following Remediation in Adult Developmental Dyslexia," *Neuron* 44(3): 411–422.

3. Timothy A. Keller and Marcel Adam Just, "Altering Cortical Connectivity: Remediation-Induced Changes in the White Matter of Poor Readers," *Neuron* 64(5): 624–631.

4. Alvaro Pascual-Leone, Nguyet Dang, Leonardo G. Cohen, Joaquim P. Brasil-Neto, Adela Cammarota, and Mark Hallett, "Modulation of Muscle Responses Evoked by Transcranial Magnetic Stimulation During the Acquisition of New Fine Motor Skills," *Journal of Neurophysiology* 74(3): 1037–1045. See also Alvaro Pascual-Leone, Amir Amedi, Felipe Fregni, and Lotfi B. Merabet, "The Plastic Human Brain Cortex," *Annual Reviews of Neuroscience* 28(2005): 377–401.

5. Adapted from personal communication with Dr. Robert Marion, April 7, 2010.

6. Kathleen Conroy, Megan Sandel, and Barry Zuckerman, "Poverty Grown Up: How Childhood Socioeconomic Status Impacts Adult Health," *Journal of Developmental and Behavioral Pediatrics* 31(2): 154–160.

7. Antoine Lutz, Heleen A. Slagter, Nancy B. Rawlings, Andrew D. Francis, Lawrence L. Greischar, and Richard J. Davidson, "Mental Training Enhances Attentional Stability: Neural and Behavioral Evidence," *Journal of Neuroscience* 29(42): 13418–13427.

8. Heleen A. Slagter, Antoine Lutz, Lawrence L. Greischar, Andrew D. Francis, Sander Nieuwenhuis, James M. Davis, and Richard J. Davidson, "Mental Training Affects Distribution of Limited Brain Resources," *PLoS Biology* 5(6): e138.

9. Ibid.

10. Lidia Zylowska, Deborah L. Ackerman, May H. Yang, Julie L. Futrell, Nancy L. Horton, T. Sigi Hale, Caroly Pataki, and Susan L. Smalley, "Mindfulness Meditation Training in Adults and Adolescents with ADHD: A Feasibility Study," *Journal of Attention Disorders*, 11(6): 737–746.

11. Lisa Flook, Susan L. Smalley, M. Jennifer Kitil, Brian M. Galla, Susan Kaiser-Greenland, Jill Locke, Erick Ishijima, and Connie Kasari, "Effects of Mindfulness Awareness Practices on Executive Functions in Elementary School Children," *Journal of Applied School Psychology* 26(1): 70–95.

12. Lisa Flook, Susan L. Smalley, M. Jennifer Kitil, Brian M. Galla, Susan Kaiser-Greenland, Jill Locke, Erick Ishijima, and Connie Kasari, "Effects of Mindfulness Awareness Practices on Executive Functions in Elementary School Children," *Journal of Applied School Psychology* 26(2010): 70–95.

13. Clancy Blair and Adele Diamond, "Biological Processes in Prevention and Intervention: The Promotion of Self-Regulation as a Means of Preventing School Failure," *Development and Psychopathology* 10(3): 899–911.

14. Adele Diamond, W. Steven Barnett, Jessica Thomas, and Sarah Munro, "Preschool Program Improves Cognitive Control," *Science* 318(5855): 1387–1388.

15. Patricia Leigh Brown, "In the Classroom, a New Focus on Quieting the Mind," *The New York Times*, June 16, 2007.

16. Sonia J. Bishop, "Trait Anxiety and Impoverished Prefrontal Control of Attention," *Nature Neuroscience* 12(1): 92–98.

Chapter 5: The Science of Mindfulness

1. Adapted from a lecture by Jennifer Bonderant, at Karme Choling, Barnet, VT, October 2008.
2. Michael S. Krasner, Ronald M. Epstein, Howard Beckman, Anthony L. Suchman, Benjamin Chapman, Christopher J. Mooney, and Timothy E. Quill, "Association of an Educational Program in Mindful Communication with Burnout, Empathy, and Attitudes Among Primary Care Physicians," *Journal of the American Medical Association* 302(12): 1284–1293.
3. Amishi P. Jha, Elizabeth A. Stanley, Anastasia Kiyonaga, Ling Wong, and Lois Gelfand, "Examining the Protective Effects of Mindfulness Training on Working Memory Capacity and Affective Experience," *Emotion* 10(1): 54–64.
4. Jon Kabat-Zinn, Elizabeth Wheeler, Timothy Light, Anne Skillings, Mark J. Scharf, Thomas G. Cropley, David Hosmer, and Jeffrey D. Bernhard, "Influence of Mindfulness Meditation-Based Stress Reduction Intervention on Rate of Skin Clearing in Patients with Moderate to Severe Psoriasis Undergoing Phototherapy (UVB) and Photochemotherapy (PUVA)," *Psychosomatic Medicine* 60(5): 625–632.
5. Richard J. Davidson, Jon Kabat-Zinn, Jessica Schumacher, Melissa Rosenkranz, Daniel Muller, Saki F. Santorelli, Ferris Urbanowski, Anne Harrington, Katherine Bonus, and John F. Sheridan, "Alterations in Brain and Immune Function Produced by Mindfulness Meditation," *Psychosomatic Medicine* 65(4): 564–570.
6. J. David Creswell, Hector F. Myers, Steven W. Cole, and Michael R. Irwin, "Mindfulness Meditation Training Effects on CD4+ T Lymphocytes in HIV-1 Infected Adults: A Small Randomized Controlled Trial," *Brain, Behavior, and Immunity* 23(2): 184–188.
7. Willem Kuyken, Sarah Byford, Rod S. Taylor, Ed Watkins, Emily Holden, Kat White, Barbara Barrett, Richard Byng, Alison Evans, Eugene Mullan, and John D. Teasdale, "Mindfulness-Based Cognitive Therapy to Prevent Relapse in Recurrent Depression," *Journal of Consulting and Clinical Psychology* 76(6): 966–978.
8. Yi-Yuan Tang, Yinghua Ma, Junhong Wang, Yaxin Fan, Shigang Feng, Qilin Lu, Qingbao Yu, Danni Sui, Mary K. Rothbart, Ming Fan, and Michale I. Posner, "Short-Term Meditation Training Improves Attention and Self-regulation," *Proceedings of the National Academy of Sciences* 103(43): 17152–17156.

9. Fadel Zeidan, Nakia S. Gordon, Junaid Merchant, and Paula Goolkasian, "The Effects of Brief Mindfulness Meditation Training on Experimentally Induced Pain," *The Journal of Pain* 11(3): 199–209.

10. Matthew D. Lieberman, Naomi I. Eisenberger, Molly J. Crockett, Sabrina M. Tom, Jennifer H. Pfeifer, and Baldwin M. Way, "Putting Feelings into Words: Affect Labeling Disrupts Amygdala Activity in Response to Affective Stimuli," *Psychological Science* 18(5): 421–428.

11. Nirbhay N. Singh, Giulio E. Lancioni, Alan S.W. Winton, Barbara C. Fisher, Robert G. Wahler, Kristen Mcaleavey, Judy Singh, and Mohamed Sabaawi, "Mindful Parenting Decreases Aggression, Noncompliance, and Self-injury in Children with Autism," *Journal of Emotional and Behavioral Disorders* 14(3): 169–177.

12. Nirbhay N. Singh, Ashvind N. Singh, Giulio E. Lancioni, Judy Singh, Alan S. W. Winton, and Angela D. Adkins, "Mindfulness Training for Parents and Their Children with ADHD Increases the Children's Compliance," *Journal of Child and Family Studies* 19(2): 157–166.

13. Richard J. Davidson, Jon Kabat-Zinn, Jessica Schumacher, Melissa Rosenkranz, Daniel Muller, Saki F. Santorelli, Ferris Urbanowski, Anne Harrington, Katherine Bonus, and John F. Sheridan, "Alterations in Brain and Immune Function Produced by Mindfulness Meditation," *Psychosomatic Medicine* 65(4): 564–570.

14. Sara W. Lazar, Catherine E. Kerr, Rachel H. Wasserman, Jeremy R. Gray, Douglas N. Greve, Michael T. Treadway, Metta McGarvey, Brian T. Quinn, Jeffery A. Dusek, Herbert Benson, Scott L. Rauch, Christopher I. Moore, and Bruce Fischl, "Meditation Experience Is Associated with Increased Cortical Thickness," *Neuroreport* 16(17): 1893–1897.

Chapter 6: Taking Care of Yourself: Mindfulness in Action

1. Kosho Ushiyama, *Opening the Hand of Thought* (Somerville, MA: Wisdom Publications, 2004).

2. Story related in various talks by Jack Kornfield, doctor of clinical psychology and founder of insight meditation.

3. CA Hutcherson, EM Seppala, and JJ Gross, "Loving-kindness meditation increases social connectedness," *Emotion* 8, no. 5 (October 2008): 720–724.

4. Antoine Lutz, Julie Brefczynski-Lewis, Tom Johnstone, and Richard J. Davidson, "Regulation of the Neural Circuitry of Emotion by Compassion Meditation: Effects of Meditative Expertise," *PLoS One* 3(3): e1897.

5. Ruth A. Baer, Gregory T. Smith, Jaclyn Hopkins, Jennifer Krietemeyer, and Leslie Toney, "Using Self-Report Assessment Methods to Explore Facets of Mindfulness," *Assessment* 13(1): 27–45.

Chapter 7: Behavior: Avoiding the "No, David" Approach

1. Hamid Alizadeh, Kimberly F. Applequist, and Frederick L. Coolidge, "Parental Self-Confidence, Parenting Styles and Corporal Punishment in Families of ADHD Children in Iran," *Child Abuse and Neglect* 31(5): 567–572.

2. H. Niederhüffer, B. Hackenberg, and K. Lanzendorfer, "Family Coherence and ADHD," *Physiological Reports*, 91(1): 123–126. See also Russell A. Barkley, *Attention-Deficit Hyperactivity Disorder: A Handbook for Diagnosis and Treatment*, 3rd ed. (New York: The Guildford Press, 2006), 195.

3. Jack Kornfield (Lecture given at "Mindfulness and Psychotherapy: Cultivating Well-being in the Present Moment," UCLA Extension and Lifespan Learning Institute, Los Angeles, CA, October 2007.)

4. Generation M^2, Media in the Lives of 8–18 Year Olds, A Kaiser Family Foundations Study, January, 2010.

5. Thomas N. Robinson, Marta L. Wilde, Lisa C. Navracruz, K. Farish Haydel, and Ann Varady, "Effects of Reducing Children's Television and Video Game Use on Aggressive Behavior: A Randomized Controlled Trial," *Archives of Pediatrics and Adolescent Medicine* 155(1): 17–23.

6. Robert Weis and Brittany C. Cerankosky, "Effects of Video-Game Ownership on Young Boys' Academic and Behavioral Functioning: A Randomized and Controlled Study," *Psychological Science* 20(18): 1–8.

7. Linda S. Pagani, Caroline Fitzpatrick, Tracie A. Barnett, and Eric Dubow, "Prospective Associations Between Early Childhood Television Exposure and Academic, Psychological and Physical Well-being by Middle Childhood," *Archives of Pediatrics and Adolescent Medicine* 164(5): 425–431. See also Madeline A. Dalton,

James D. Sargent, Michael L. Beach, Linda Titus-Ernstoff, Jennifer J. Gibson, M. Bridget Ahrens, Jennifer J. Tickle, and Todd F. Heatherton, "Effect of Viewing Smoking in Movies on Adolescent Smoking Initiation: A Cohort Study," *Lancet* 362(9380): 281–285.

8. Heather L. Kirkorian, Tiffany A. Pempek, Lauren A. Murphy, Marie E. Schmidt, and Daniel R. Anderson, "The Impact of Background Television on Parent-Child Interaction," *Child Development* 80(5): 1350–1359.

9. Linda S. Pagani, Caroline Fitzpatrick, Tracie A. Barnett, and Eric Dubow, "Prospective Associations Between Early Childhood Television Exposure and Academic, Psychological and Physical Well-being by Middle Childhood," *Archives of Pediatrics and Adolescent Medicine* 164(5): 425–431.

10. Frederick J. Zimmerman and Dimitri A. Christakis, "Associations Between Content Types of Early Media Exposure and Subsequent Attentional Problems," *Pediatrics* 120(5): 986–992; Edward L. Swing, Douglas A. Gentile, Craig A. Anderson, and David A. Walsh, *Pediatrics*, published online July 5, 2010.

11. Chih-Hung Ko, Ju-Yu Yen, Cheng-Sheng Chen, Yi-Chun Yeh, and Cheng-Fang Yen, "Predictive Values of Psychiatric Symptoms for Internet Addiction in Adolescents: A Two-Year Prospective Study," *Archives of Pediatrics and Adolescent Medicine* 163(10): 937–943.

12. Josephine Elia, Paul Ambrosini, and Wade Berrettini, "ADHD Characteristics: I. Concurrent Co-Morbidity Patterns in Children and Adolescents," *Child and Adolescent Psychiatry and Mental Health* 2(1): 15.

Chapter 8: Education: Rallying the Team

1. Patricia N. Pastor and Cynthia N. Reuben, "Diagnosed Attention Deficit Hyperactivity Disorder and Learning Disability: United States, 2004–2006," National Center for Health Statistics, *Vital Health Statistics* 10(237).

2. Joshua Langberg, Jeffery N. Epstein, Christina M. Urbanowicz, John O. Simon, and Amanda J. Graham, "Efficacy of an Organization Skills Intervention to Improve the Academic Functioning of Students with Attention-Deficit/Hyperactivity Disorder," *School Psychology Quarterly* 23(3): 407–417.

3. National Reading Panel, "Teaching Children to Read: An Evidence-Based Assessment of the Scientific Research Literature on Reading and Its Implications for Reading Instruction ," U.S. Department of Health and Human Services Public Health Service National Institutes of Health National Institute of Child Health and Human Development NIH Pub. No. 00–4769 April 2000

4. Michael L. Bloomquist, Gerald J. August, and Risk Ostrander, "Effects of a School-Based Cognitive-Behavioral Intervention for ADHD Children," *Journal of Abnormal Child Psychology* 19(5): 591–605.

5. Nigel Hastings and Joshua Schwieso, "Tasks and Tables: The Effects of Seating Arrangements on Task Engagement in Primary Classrooms," *Educational Research* 37(3): 279–291.

6. Susan Shur-Fen Gau, Chui-De Chiu, Chi-Yung Shang, Andrew Tai-Ann Cheng, and Wei-Tsuen Soong, "Executive Function in Adolescence Among Children with Attention-Deficit/Hyperactivity Disorder in Taiwan," *Journal of Developmental and Behavioral Pediatrics* 30(6): 525–534.

Chapter 9: Medical Options for ADHD

1. The MTA Cooperative Group, "A 14-Month Randomized Clinical Trial of Treatment Strategies for Attention-Deficit/Hyperactivity Disorder," *Archives of General Psychiatry* 56(12): 1073–1086.

2. Kerstin Konrad, Susanne Neufang, Gereon R. Fink, and Beate Herpertz-Dahlmann, "Long-Term Effects of Methylphenidate on Neural Networks Associated with Executive Attention in Children with ADHD: Results from a Longitudinal Functional MRI Study," *Journal of the American Academy of Child and Adolescent Psychiatry* 46(12): 1633–1641.

3. Robyn L. Powers, David J. Marks, Carlin J. Miller, Jeffrey H. Newcorn, and Jeffrey M. Halperin, "Stimulant Treatment in Children with ADHD Moderates Adolescent Academic Outcome," *Journal of Child and Adolescent Psychopharmacology* 18(5): 449–459.

4. Margaret Semrud-Clikeman, Steven Pliszka, and Mario Liotti, "Executive Functioning in Children with Attention-Deficit/Hyperactivity Disorder: Combined Type with or without a Stimulant Medication History," *Neuropsychology* 22(3): 329–340.

5. Joseph Biederman, Michael C. Monuteaux, Thomas Spencer, Timothy E. Wilens, and Stephen V. Faraone, "Do Stimulants Protect Against

Psychiatric Disorders in Youth with ADHD? A 10-Year Follow-Up Study," *Pediatrics* 124(1): 71–78.

6. Russell A. Barkley, et al., "International Consensus Statement on ADHD," *Clinical Child and Family Psychology Review* 5(2): 89–111.

7. T. E. Wilens, J. Adamson, M. C. Monuteaux, S. V. Faraone, M. Schillinger, D. Westerberg, and J. Biederman, "Effect of Prior Stimulant Treatment for Attention-Deficit/Hyperactivity Disorder on Subsequent Risk for Cigarette Smoking and Alcohol and Drug Use Disorders in Adolescents," *Archives of Pediatrics and Adolescent Medicine* 162(10): 916–921.

8. Russell A. Barkley, et al., "International Consensus Statement on ADHD," *Clinical Child and Family Psychology Review* 5(2): 89–111.

9. Brendan F. Andrade, Darlene A. Brodeur, Daniel A. Waschbusch, Sherry H. Stewart, and Robin McGee, "Selective and Sustained Attention as Predictors of Social Problems in Children with Typical and Disordered Attention Abilities," *Journal of Attention Disorders* 12(4): 341–352.

10. Russell A. Barkley, et al., "International Consensus Statement on ADHD," *Clinical Child and Family Psychology Review* 5(2): 89–111.

11. Cynthia L. Liebson, Slavica K. Katusic, William J. Barbaresi, Jeanine Ransom, and Peter C. O'Brien, "Use and Costs of Medical Care for Children and Adolescents with and without Attention-Deficit/Hyperactivity Disorder, *Journal of the American Medical Association* 285(1): 60–66. See also Andrine R. Swensen, Howard G. Birnbaum, Kristina Secnik, Maryna Marynchenko, Paul Greenberg, and Ami Claxton, "Attention-Deficit/Hyperactivity Disorder: Increased Costs for Patients and Their Families," *Journal of the American Academy of Child and Adolescent Psychiatry* 42(12): 1415–1423.

12. Evelyne Touchette, Sylvana M. Cote, Dominique Petit, Xuecheng Liu, Michel Boivin, Bruno Falissard, Richard E. Tremblay, and Jacques Y. Montplaisir, "Short Nighttime Sleep-Duration and Hyperactivity Trajectories in Early Childhood," *Pediatrics* 124(5): e985–993.

13. Joseph Biederman, MD, Thomas J Spencer, MD, Michale C. Monuteaux, ScD, and Stephen V. Faraone, PhD, "A Naturalistic 10-Year Prospective Study of Height and Weight Children with Attention Deficit/Hyperactivity Disorder Grown Up: Sex and Treatment Effects, *The Journal of Pediatrics,* published online June 7, 2010.

14. Thomas J. Spencer, Stephen V. Faraone, Joseph Biederman, Marc Lerner, Kimberly M. Cooper, Brenda Zimmerman, and Concerta Study Group, "Does Prolonged Therapy with a Long-acting Stimulant Suppress Growth in Children with ADHD?" *Journal of the American Academy of Child and Adolescent Psychiatry* 45(5): 527–537. See also Ran D. Goldman, "ADHD Stimulants and Their Effect on Height in Children," *Canadian Family Physician* 56 (February 2010): 145–146.

15. Suzanne McCarthy, Noel Cranswick, Laura Potts, Eric Taylor, Ian Wong, "Mortality associated with attention-deficit hyperactivity disorder (ADHD) drug treatment: a retrospective cohort study of children, adolescents and young adults using the general practice research database," *Drug Safety*, 2009; 32(11):1089–1096; Amut G.Winterstein, Tobias Gerhard, Jonathan Shuster, Michael Johnson, Julie M. Zito and Arwa Saidi, "Cardiac Safety of Central Nervous System Stimulants in Children and Adolescents with Attention Deficit/Hyperactivity Disorder." *Pediatrics*, 2007; 120; e1494–1501.

16. Russell A. Barkley, "Sudden Death and Stimulant Treatment: Is There a Relationship?" *The ADHD Report*, 17(4): 1–4.

17. Veit Roessner, Monika Robatzek, Guido Knapp, Tobias Banaschewski, and Aribert Rothenberger, "First-onset Tics in Patients with Attention-Deficit-Hyperactivity Disorder: Impact of Stimulants," *Developmental Medicine and Child Neurology* 48(7): 616–621.

18. Mark L. Wolraich, David B. Wilson, and J. Wade White, "The Effect of Sugar on Behavior or Cognition in Children: A Meta-analysis," *Journal of the American Medical Association* 27(20): 1617–1621.

19. Donna McCann, Angelina Barrett, Alison Cooper, Debbie Crumpler, Lindy Dalen, Kate Grimshaw, Elizabeth Kitchin, Kris Lok, Lucy Porteous, Emily Prince, Edmund Sonuga-Barke, John O. Warner, and Jim Stevenson, "Food Additives and Hyperactive Behavior in 3-Year-Old and 8/9-Year-Old Children in the Community: A Randomized, Double-Blinded, Placebo-Controlled Trial," *Lancet* 370(9598): 1560–1567.

20. Lisa Flook, Susan L. Smalley, M. Jennifer Kitil, Brian M. Galla, Susan Kaiser-Greenland, Jill Locke, Eric Ishijima, and Connie Kasari, "Effects of Mindful Awareness Practices on Executive Functions in Elementary School Children," *Journal of Applied School Psychology*, 26(1): 70–95.

21. Holger Gevensleben, Birgit Holl, Bjorn Albrecht, Claudia Vogel, Dieter Schlamp, Oliver Kratz, Petra Studer, Aribert Rothenberger, Gunther Moll, and Hartmut Heinrich, "Is Neurofeedback an

Efficacious Treatment for ADHD? A Randomized Controlled Clinical Trial," *Journal of Child Psychology and Psychiatry* 50(7): 780–789. See also Torkel Klingberg, Elisabeth Fernell, Pernille J. Olesen, Mats Johnson, Per Gustafsson, Kerstin Dahlstrom, Christopher G. Gillberg, Hans Forssberg, and Helena Westerberg, "Computerized Training of Working Memory in Children with ADHD: A Randomized, Controlled Trial," *Journal of the American Academy of Child and Adolescent Psychiatry* 44(2): 177–186.

22. Romina M. Barros, Ellen J. Silver, and Ruth E. K. Stein, "School Recess and Group Classroom Behavior," *Pediatrics* 123(2): 431–436.

23. Andrea Faber Taylor and Frances E. Kuo, "Children with Attention Deficits Concentrate Better after Walk in the Park," *Journal of Attention Disorders* 12(5): 402–409.

Index

504 plan, 163–5, 169

"ABC" approach, 151
absence seizures, 32
academic accommodations for ADHD, 173
acting out, 9, 16, 61, 119
ADD, *See* attention deficit disorder
Adderall, 184
Adderall XR, 184
ADHD, *See* attention deficit hyperactivity disorder
ADHD checklists, *See* checklists
ADHD medications, *See* medications list
ADHD subtypes, *See* subtypes
adult approval, 57–8, 131
adult attention, 57–8
advertising, avoiding, 147–9
aggressive behavior, and media, 147–8
alcohol use, 146–7, 182
alternative treatments, 3, 194–8
    attention training, 195–6
    auditory and vision training, 196–7
    computer training, 196
    dietary changes, 194–5
    exercise, 196
    guidelines in, 197–8
Alzheimer's disease, 77
American Academy of Pediatrics, 148
amygdala, 63, 77–9
antidepressants, 185–6
anxiety
    and ADHD, 32
    and attention, 64–5
    disorders, *See* anxiety disorders
    and managing behavior, 129
    and mindfulness, 76
anxiety disorders, 32, 35, 76

atomoxitine, 185–6
attention deficit disorder (ADD), 10
attention deficit hyperactivity disorder
        (ADHD)
    and the brain, *See* frontal lobes
    checklists for, *See* checklists
    defining, 10–12
    diagnosing, *See* diagnosis of ADHD
    and early intervention, 26, 33, 36–7, 109
    foundations in care, 120–1, 177–8
    as genetic, 11–12, 55
    outgrowing, 25–6, 47
    and parenting, *See* parenting; parenting
        guidelines
    and personality, *See* personality
    and politics, 9–11
    proactive plan for, 19–20
    reality of, *See* reality of ADHD
    reframing, 47–8
    subtypes of, *See* subtypes of ADHD
    symptoms of, *See* symptoms of ADHD
    treatment, *See* medical options
attention management, and ADHD, 41–2, 168
    in the classroom, 168
attention shifting, 51, 56, 108, 143
attention training, 2–3, 51–70, 88–91, 195–6
    and ADHD, 55–7, 195–6
    as alternative treatment, 195–6
    and anxiety, 64–5
    as brain training, 52–3
    and genes, 54–5
    and judgment, 61–3
    and meditation, 55–7, 65–70
    mindfulness meditation, 67–9
    and mirroring behavior, 57–8
    and parenting, 88–91
    neuroplasticity, 52–4

attention training—*Continued*
    and stress management, 2–3, 60–1, 63–70
    and teaching children to focus, 58–60
"attentional blink," 56
"auditory processing disorder," 35–6
auditory training, 196–7
autism, 23, 35–6, 76
autistic spectrum disorder, 35

background television, 149
"bad" behavior, 10, 14–15, 29, 45, 92, 126, 135
Barkley, Russell, 16, 150
bed time, *See* sleep habits
behavioral planning, 13–14, 166–7
being different, child's awareness of, 15–17, 47
"best self," 178–9
biology, and ADHD, 4, 10–12, 15–18,
            21–2, 41, 44–5, 51, 55, 98, 120,
            126, 140, 151, 177, 201–2
bipolar disorder, 32
body scan, 82–3, 117
borderline personality disorder, 71, 75
brain benefits of meditation, 76–8
brain growth/connectivity
    See neuroplasticity
brain manager, 12–13, 39–47, 157–60
    See frontal lobe
breathing meditation, 2, 67–9, 84–5, 100
Brown ADHD scales, 30
Buddhism, 72
burnout, 3, 73

caffeine, 79
checklists for ADHD
    communication, 110
    diagnosis, 29–30
    executive function symptoms, 40–7
    homework, 171–3
    subtype symptoms, 27
    symptoms of ADHD, 27, 40–7
    management of ADHD, 203–5
children with ADHD
    See personality; self-awareness; self-esteem;
    social relationships
child development
    and media, 147
    typical, 23–5
chronic anemia, 32
cigarette smoking, 55, 85, 147
classroom tips, 167–9
    See education

Clonidine, 184
cognitive flexibility, 58–60, 203
combined type (ADHD), 10, 26–7
commercials, 147–9
common medications for ADHD, 184–6
communication
    with adults, 108–10
    checklist, 110
    with children, 105–8
    with the school, 164–5
comorbid conditions, 34–5
compassion, 48, 98–105, 108, 112, 115–16,
            118–19, 128, 145, 150, 152, 195, 205
computer guidelines, 146–50
computer training (alternative treatment), 196
conduct disorders, 34–5
confidence building, 14, 28, 43, 48, 131, 159
    See self-esteem
Conners checklist, 30
consequences, 25, 137–40
    calm, 138–40
    immediate, 25, 137–40
    See time out
consistency, parental, 14–15, 128, 133–6,
            141–2, 153, 201, 204
    and oppositional behavior, 153
    and routine, 133–5
    self-monitoring, 135–6
conversation meditation, 109–10
corrections, constant, 116, 125, 130–3,
            136, 162
cortex, 77
cortisol, 61, 76
creativity
    and ADHD, 180
    and parenting, 17, 110–11, 128–30, 144

danger to themselves, *See* self-
            endangerment
daydreaming, 13, 24, 29, 32–3, 42, 91, 158,
            160, 174
Daytrana, 184
decisions, 110–13
delayed gratification, 59, 142, 146, 148
depression, 3, 17–18, 32, 71, 75–6, 129,
            181, 186, 197
developmental delays, 23, 33–4
Dexidrine, 184
diagnosis of ADHD, 21–37
    and age, 28–9, 30–1
    clinical diagnosis, 21–3, 26–34

and comorbid conditions, 34–5
and early intervention, 26, 33, 36–7, 109
four steps toward, 29–33
and over-diagnosis, 21–2
and "impairment," 20, 33
and objectivity, 24–5, 36–7
and other medical conditions, 31–2, 34–5
outgrowing, 25–6
and multiple settings, 26, 29, 30
and persistence of symptoms, 29, 30–1
and rating scales, 30
and school psychologists, 23
and second opinion, 23
and subtypes, 26–9
and terminology, 35–6
and testing, 34
Diamond, Adele, 60
dietary changes, 194–5
differential diagnosis, 31
discernment, 93
disciplining, *See* parenting guidelines
distractibility, 13, 15, 22, 29, 32, 42, 44,
        108, 133, 138, 143, 160, 163,
        178–80, 183, 191–2, 201
dysgraphia, 161
dyslexia, 54

early diagnosis, 28–9
early intervention, 26, 33, 36–7, 109
eating meditation, 91–2
education of children with ADHD, 17,
        42–6, 157–76, 193, 202, 204
    academic accommodations, 173
    academic picture, 160–2
    and adaptations, 166–7
    and adjustments, 174–6
    behavioral planning, 166–7
    and the brain manager, 157–60
    challenges in, 42–6
    and curricula, 161–2
    classroom supports, 167–9
    effort and motivation, 43–4
    and executive function skills, 42–6
    homework support, 170–3
    and medication, 193
    organizational supports, 167–9
    and parents' rights, 162–4
    school communication, 164–5
    and scientific methods, 161–2
    task management, 42–3
    and teacher expectations, 167

testing, 169–70
and working memory, 45–6
See grading; mathematics; reading
        comprehension
effort and motivation, 43–4
electroencephalogram (EEG), 196
emotional regulation, 13, 40, 44–5,
        74, 77
empathy, 73, 101–5
evidence-based practices, 3–4, 54, 71,
        73–6, 125, 161–2, 204
executive function skills, 12–13, 39–47,
        157–60
    attention management, 41–2
    effort and motivation, 43–4
    emotional regulation, 44–5
    and education, 157–60
    self-monitoring, 46–7
    task management, 42–3
    working memory, 45–6
exercise
    and ADHD, 196
    and stress, 79
expectations
    and consistency, 136
    parenting, and ADHD, 143
    and stress, 77–9
    teacher, 167
experiencing the moment, 91–2
expert help, 21–3, 130, 145–6, 153, 205
    in diagnosis, 22–3
    and oppositional behavior, 153
    reaching out for, 130, 145–6

family life, 4, 13–14, 19, 76, 143–5, 149,
        197, 201–5
    and alternative medicine, 197
    challenges for, 13–14
    and mindfulness, 4, 19, 76
    and routine, 143–5
    support for, 201–5
fear, 54, 63–5, 77–81, 93–4, 97–8, 159
    and ADHD, 81
    and attention, 54, 63–5
    and change, 97–8
    and education, 159
    and stress, 63, 77–81, 93–4
fetal alcohol exposure, 12, 55
fight-or-flight response, 63, 77–8
Focalin, 185
Focalin XR, 185

focus, and ADHD
   and attention management, 41–2
   growth stages of, 24
   and mindfulness, 19–20
   teaching children, 58–60
food dyes, 194
forgetfulness, 22, 25, 29, 33, 36, 40, 45–6,
        101, 128, 134–5, 139, 141, 144,
        157, 163, 179, 192
   See working memory
foundations of ADHD care, 120–1, 177–8
free play, 53, 59–60, 195, 203
frontal lobe, 12–13, 25–6, 33, 35, 39–47,
        77, 126, 141–2, 157–61, 177,
        179–80, 185
   as "brain manager," 39–40, 157–60
   decreased activity of, 12–13, 35, 40
   development of, 25–6
   and developmental delays, 33
   and education, 157–60
   and learning from mistakes, 46
   and motor skills, 46–7
   and parents, 141
   skills of, 41–7
   and teenagers, 141
   and well-being, 77
   See executive function skills

gender, and ADHD, 24–5, 21, 23, 24–5
genes, 11–12, 25, 52–5, 128
   and ADHD, 11–12, 25, 128
   changing, 54–5
   and destiny, 52
gluten-free diet, 195
good judgment, 92–5
grading, 163, 170, 173, 179
guanfacine/Tenex, 185–6
guidelines,
   for basic parenting, 130–142
   for homework support, 171–173
   for media use, 148–150
   for monitoring and adjusting
      medications, 192–194
   for oppositional behaviors, 151–153

handwriting, 47, 161, 169–70, 173, 181
health and well-being, 71, 73–7
Healthy Sleep Habits, Happy Child
      (Weissbluth), 134
height, and medication, 189
helpful checklists, *See* checklists

hitting, 25, 45–6, 60, 136–7, 141
homework support, 170–3
hyperactive/impulsive type (ADHD), 10, 26–8
   symptoms checklist, 27

ignoring what you can, 136–7
individualized educational program (IEP),
      163–5
impairment, 33
impulsive type of ADHD, *See* hyperactive/
      impulsive type
impulsiveness/impulsivity
   checklist for symptoms, 27
   outgrowing, 25–6
   and parents, 15–16
   in teenagers, 25–6, 141
inattentive type (ADHD), 10, 26–9, 32
   and anxiety disorders, 32
   symptoms checklist, 27
injuries/accidents, 28, 181, 183
insomnia, 75
insula, 77
Internet, 149–50
interrupting, 27, 47, 108
intervention, 26, 33, 36–7, 109, 120–1, 177–99
   early, 26, 33, 36–7, 109
   and foundations of ADHD care, 120–1,
      177–8
   and mindfulness, 198–9
   See alternative treatments; medical options
Intuniv (guanfacine extended release), 184–5

Jha, Amishi, 73
Journal of the American Medical Association
      (JAMA), 73
judgment, 3, 61–4, 92–101
   and change, 97–8
   and compassion, 98–101
   good judgment, 92–5
   letting go of, 3, 61–4, 92–5
   practice pausing, 96–7

Kaiser-Greenland, Susan, 196
know your child, 140–1

language delays, 35, 147
lead toxicity, 12, 32
learning disability, 21, 23, 31, 34–5, 158,
      161, 163, 197
letting go, 3, 61–4, 92–8
   of judgment, 3, 61–4, 92–5

practice, 97–8
stop and let go, 98
limits, 14–15, 45, 59, 125, 128, 135, 141,
     146, 148–9, 153, 201, 204
   and consistency, 128, 141, 153, 201, 204
   and emotional regulation, 45
   media, 146, 148–9
   as teaching tool, 135
   upholding, 153
   value of setting, 14–15
lists, 133–4, 158–9
lovingkindness, 103–5
Lutz, Antoine, 56

magnetic resonance imaging (MRI), 54, 76
management
   bed time, 134
   checklist, 203–5
   media, 146–50
   medication, 190–4
   of oppositional behavior, 150–3
   of yourself, 46–7, 152–5
management checklist (ADHD), 203–5
marriage, and ADHD, 1, 18, 129–30
mathematics, 37, 44, 53, 60, 63, 160–2, 181
media management, 146–50
medical options, 177–99
   child's perspective, 178–9
   medication, See medications
   and research, 180–1
medications, 179–94, 202, 204
   and "best self," 178–9
   child's perspective on, 178–9
   choosing, 184–6
   and creativity, 180
   facts about, 179–80
   and family life, 202
   guidelines, 192–4
   list of, 184–6
   managing, 190–4
   myths of, 10, 181–2
   and "rebound," 188
   research about, 180–1
   risks and benefits, 182–4
   side effects, 186–93
   and substance abuse, 182
   types of, 184–6
   See stimulants
medications list, 184–6
meditation, 2–3, 19, 55–60, 65–70, 71–2,
     74, 76–7, 82–5, 89–92, 100,

103–5, 109–10, 112–14, 117–20,
     154–5, 174–6, 181, 195, 205
   and attention, 19, 55–7, 65–70, 195
   basic, 2–3, 67–70
   benefits of, 55–6, 71–2, 74, 77, 85
   and the breath, 100, 175
   and clarity, 112–14
   and the cortex, 77
   and mental habits, 174–6
   and oppositional behaviors, 181
   types of, See meditation types
   See mindfulness-based stress
      reduction (MBSR)
   meditation types, See conversation
      meditation; eating
   meditation; metta; mindfulness meditation;
      walking meditation; breathing
      meditation; stop and let go (STOP)
mental distraction, and parenting, 66, 151–2
mental habits, and meditation, 174–6
mental health issues, and ADHD, 21, 23,
     31–2, 34, 188–9
Metadate CD/ER, 184
Methylin, 184
metta (or lovingkindness), 103–5
The Mindful Child (Kaiser-Greenland), 196
mindfulness, 2–4, 19–20, 60, 65–70, 71–85,
     113–20, 195, 198–9, 202, 205
   brain benefits of, 76–7
   defined, 19–20
   expectations and stress, 77–9
   and health and well-being, 73–6
   in action, See mindfulness in action
   instructions to begin, 67–9
   life benefits of, 2–4
   and medical intervention, 198–9
   new perspective on, 71–3
   science of, 71–85
   tools for everyday life, 113–20
mindfulness in action, 87–121
   and ADHD, 101–5, 120–2
   and communication, 105–10
   compassion, 98–105
   decisions, 110–13
   direct your attention, 89–91
   everyday tools for, 113–20
   experience the moment, 91–2
   good judgment, 92–5
   letting go, 97–8
   practice pausing, 96–7
   six-week program for, 116–20

mindfulness in action—*Continued*
  stepping into life, 88–9
mindfulness-based cognitive therapy for
      depression (MBCT), 75–6
mindfulness-based stress reduction
      (MBSR), 2–3, 71–2, 84
mindfulness meditation, 56, 65, 67–9,
      71–5, 89–90
  example of, 67–9
  and physical ailments, 74–5
mirror neurons, 57–8, 61
modeling behavior, 57–9, 61, 97, 119, 130,
      140, 148–9, 153, 195
mood swings, 32, 44
motivation, 4, 40–1, 43–4, 102, 111,
      115–16, 126, 133, 135, 141, 159,
      170, 172–3, 202
  academic, 141, 159, 170, 172–3
  and achievement, 126
  external, 43–4
  maintaining, 135
  struggles, 40
  See rewards
motor skills, 24, 46–7, 161
moving about, and health (parental), 154–5
multi-tasking, myth of, 84
Multimodal Treatment of ADHD (MTA),
      180–1
multiple settings, and symptoms, 26, 29, 30

narrative writing, 45, 160–1
negativity bias, 94–5
neurofeedback, 196
neuroplasticity, 26, 51–4
No, David! (Shannon), 130
"No, David!" trap, 130–3
non-stimulants, 185
Nortriptyline (and other anti-depressants), 184
note-taking, 161, 173
nutritional deficiencies, 195

obesity, 147, 149
objectivity, 24–5, 36–7, 112, 129, 152, 183,
      198–9, 202, 204
oppositional behavior, 34, 146, 150–3, 181
  and ADHD, 34
  guidelines for, 151–3
  managing, 150–3
  and medication, 181
  and therapy, 146

oppositional disorder, 150
organizational challenges, 4, 13, 22, 25–6,
      29, 40, 42–3, 115, 126, 128, 158,
      161, 166–70, 173
  classroom support for, 167–9
  and homework, 170
  and task management, 42–3
organizational skills, 161, 167–70, 173
outgrowing ADHD, 25–6, 47
over-diagnosis, illusion of, 21–2
overeating, 40, 46, 80

parenting, and ADHD
  and anxiety and depression, 17–18, 129
  and attention training, 88–91
  and biology, 55
  and brain development, 53
  change begins with you, 126–30
  challenges of, 1–2, 3–4, 9–10, 13–20,
      129, 203–5
  checklists for, *See* checklists
  and creativity, 17, 110–11, 128–30, 144
  and diagnosis, *See* diagnosis
  guidelines for, *See* parenting guidelines
  and objectivity, 25, 36
  and open-mindedness, 13–15, 62
  and marriage, *See* marriage
  and media, *See* media management
  and mindfulness, 1–4, 19–20, 58–60, 76
      See mindfulness in action
  myths of, 17–19
  and proactive plan, 19–20
  and reaching out, 130
  scheduled time with children, 57–8,
      150, 152
  and terminology, 35–6
  See modeling behavior; stress
      management
parenting guidelines, 130–45
  consequences, 137–40
  consistency, *See* consistency
  and family life, 143–5
  ignoring what you can, 136–7
  know your child, 140–1
  and limits, *See* limits
  media management, 146–50
  and oppositional behavior, 150–3
  and perspective, 141–2
  praise and reward, 130–3
  routine, 133–5

therapy, 145–6
See checklists
parenting style, 125–30
parents with ADHD, 25, 128
pausing, *See* practice pausing
pediatricians, 10, 22, 36, 162, 189, 191
personality, and ADHD, 15–17, 28, 33
perspective, maintaining, 141–2
play-based activities, 59–60
point of view exercise, 145
politics of ADHD, 9–11
positive feedback, 28, 97, 107, 125, 130–1,
        135, 142, 204
practice pausing, 96–7, 152–3
praise, 125, 127–8, 130–3, 135, 137, 152,
        166, 184, 202, 204
    emphasizing, 125, 127–8, 130–3
    and rewards, 130–3, 202, 204
premature birth, 12
preschoolers, 15, 23–4, 28, 58–60, 138
problem solving, 4, 19, 46, 59, 74, 78–9,
        81, 90, 110, 128, 135–6, 140, 144,
        150, 169, 176, 195
procrastination, 33, 43
professional help, *See* expert help
psoriasis, 74

rating scales, 30
reaching out for help, 130, 145–6
    See expert help
reactivity, 79–83
reading comprehension, 45, 54, 158,
        160–2, 174, 178, 180–1
reality of ADHD, 1–2, 9–11, 15–19, 22, 55
    See biology, and ADHD
"rebound," 188
Rehabilitation Act of 1974, 163
respond, not react, 79–83
reward system, 131–3, 135, 141–2, 144,
        167, 172, 201
    building, 132–3
    and routine, 135
rewards, 40–1, 43–5, 121, 127, 130–3, 135, 141–2,
        144, 150, 153, 166–7, 172, 202, 204
    building reward system, 132–3
    and education, 43–4, 172
    and motivation, 43–5, 172
    and praise, 130–3, 202, 204
Ritalin (methylphenidate), 184
Ritalin LA, 184

routine, the power of, 133–5
ruminating, 2, 19, 64, 66–7, 75–6, 80–2,
        88, 97, 100, 114–15, 150, 152, 174

Saltzman, Amy, 116–17
scheduled time with children, 57–8, 150, 152
school, *See* education
school psychologists, 23
second opinion, 23
self-awareness, 15–17, 47
self-endangerment, 24–5, 28, 33, 55, 136–7
self-esteem, 14, 19, 28–9, 126, 131, 133,
        146, 191, 202
self-doubt, 94–5, 99–100
self-monitoring
    and ADHD, 13, 25, 41, 46–7, 160, 180,
        187
    parental, 135–6, 152
self-regulation, 4, 13, 39, 58–60, 111, 116,
        120, 135, 174, 179–80, 184–5,
        187, 195, 198
"sensory integration disorder," 35
"should," 13–14, 16, 40–1, 58, 61–4, 66, 79–80,
        88, 93–6, 99, 112, 115–17, 126
"shouldn't," 61, 64, 93, 95–6, 116
side effects (of medication), 186–93
sitting still, 15, 24, 35–6, 137, 151, 154,
        157–8
six-week program for mindfulness, 116–20
sleep habits, 134, 142
sleep problems, 32, 35, 79, 134, 187
skillful communication, *See* communication
SNAP checklist, 30
social media, 149
social relationships (and ADHD), 13–14,
        17–18, 22, 24–5, 27, 33, 44, 47,
        108, 191–2
    growth stages of, 24
    and imaginative play time, 24, 33
    and inattentive-type symptoms, 22
    and interrupting, 27, 47, 108
    and mood swings, 44
    standing too close, 18, 47
    talking too loud, 47
spending time with your children, 57–8,
        150, 152
"staring spells," 32
statistics on ADHD, 11–12
stimulants, 184–91
stomach upset, and medication, 187

stop and let go (STOP), 98
Strattera (atomoxitine), 184
strengths of child, 15–17, 28, 135
stress, and learning, 53, 55, 74
stress cycles, 61, 65–70, 78–83, 135
    See body scan
stress hormones, 61, 63–4, 76
stress management, 2–5, 60–70, 71–85,
        92–5, 129
    attention and anxiety, 64–5
    breaking stress cycles, 65–70, 79–83
    and expectations, 77–9
    letting go of judgment, 61–4, 92–5
    and mindfulness, 2–5, 71–85
    and open-mindedness, 62–3
    respond, not react, 79–83
    and self-doubt, 94–5
strict environments, 125–6
substance abuse, 146–7, 181–2
subtypes of ADHD, 10, 26–9
    checklist for, 27
    See combined type; hyperactive/
        impulsive type;
    inattentive type
sugar, 194
symptoms of ADHD, 26–33, 40–7
    checklists for, 27, 40–7
    clinical, 26–33, 40–7
    and "impairment," 33
    in multiple settings, 30
    and other medical conditions, 31–2
    persistence of, 29, 30–1
    and subtypes, 26–9
    See executive function skills
symptoms checklists, 27, 40–7

tai chi, 72, 154
taking time for yourself, 83–5
task management, 42–3
teacher expectations, 167
teaching children to focus, 58–60
teenagers, 25–6, 141, 146, 148–50, 153,
        170, 181, 183

    and behavior modification, 153
    and electronic media, 146, 148–50
    and family time, 149
    and handwriting, 170
    and impulsivity, 25–6, 141
    and stimulants, 181
    and substance abuse, 181, 183
television guidelines, 146–50
Tenex / guanfacine, 184–5
terminology, 35–6
test-taking, 161, 169–70, 173
testing, and diagnosis, 34
texting, 148–9
therapy, 145–6
thyroid disease, 31–2
tic disorders, 35, 185–6, 189–90
time distortion, and ADHD, 47
time management, 13, 40, 161, 169
time out, 139, 141–2, 147
token economies, See reward system
treatment for ADHD, See intervention
typical development, See child
        development, typical

Vanderbilt checklist, 30
vision training, 196–7
Vyvanse, 184

Weissbluth, Marc, 134
walking meditation, 154–5
weight loss, and medication, 186–90, 192
well-being, 3, 14, 17, 58–9, 65, 70, 71–7,
        102, 113, 115, 119–20, 202, 204
Wellbutrin, 184, 186
Western medicine, 3, 71–6
working memory, 45–6, 60, 133, 160, 170,
        196
writing, 45, 160–1

yoga, 58–9, 72, 119, 154–5, 195

Zinn, Jon Kabat, 71–2, 74
Zylowska, Lidia, 56–7